GLUCUT COACHING

GLUCUTCOACHING

Japanese Lifestyle for Diabetes Prevention
based on the 500 Calorie Meal

Hector Hocsman

自然

DISCLAIMER: GLUCUT COACHING is a self-managed, lifestyle coaching program, not a replacement for medical care. The GLUCUT COACHING program supports education, data management, motivation, and behavior modification habits that will not compromise the advice of your healthcare provider.

If you have been diagnosed with Obesity , pre-diabetes or type 2 diabetes, continue to get professional medical advice from your professional healthcare provider. Your healthcare team is essential. They understand the human body and will assist you with your medication, activity levels, temperature levels, emotional stress, and all other factors that contribute to your wellbeing. Although following the GLUCUT COACHING program may improve your physical state enough that you can reduce your medications, always check with your healthcare provider before making changes to your treatment, medication regimen, or activity levels.

The information in this document is generic and not specific to any single individual. It offers a summary of information that raises awareness of specific conditions and behaviors. It does not advocate for a specific treatment or change.

Published in the United States by GLUCUT LLC, GLUCUT COACHING, a United States Registered TM company.

www. glucut.com

ISBN-13: 978-0-6924-6656-8
ISBN-10: 0-6924-6656-8

Book design and layout by Ellene Glenn Moore
Cover and logo design by Hector Hocsman

THIS BOOK IS DEDICATED TO EISUKE ITO, 76

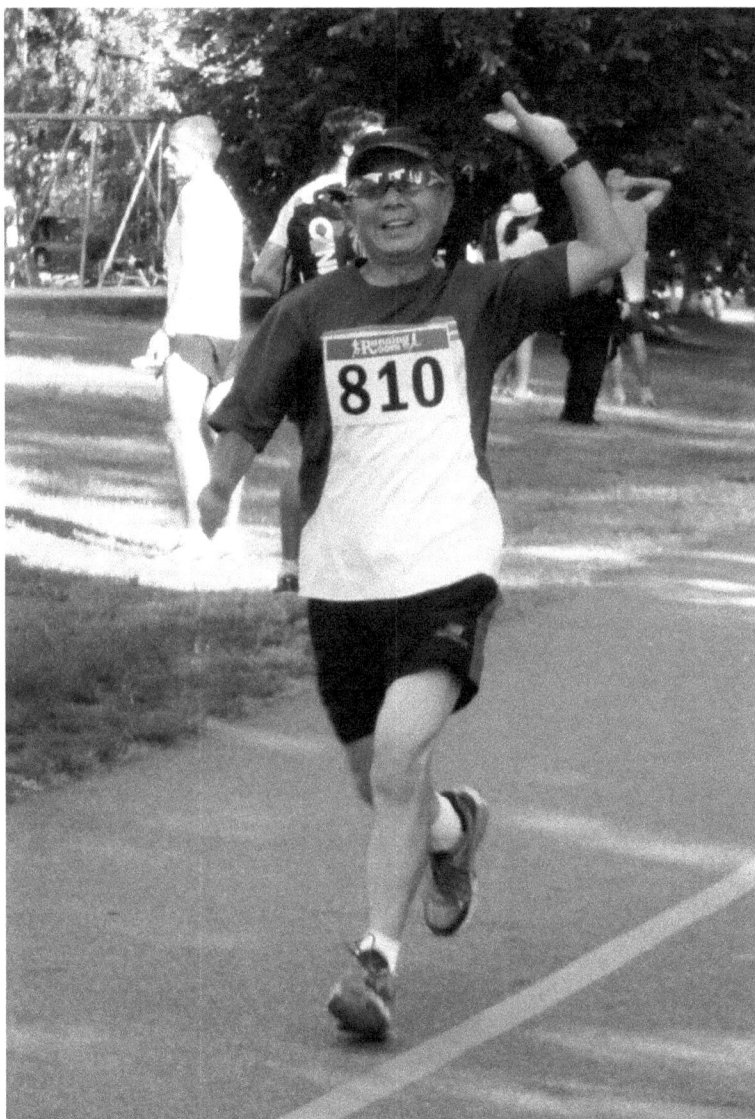

Vancouver, 2013 Marathon

CONTENTS

D. MONITORING SYSTEM   101

A PERSONAL NOTE ON MOTIVATION

While creating this program, I encountered a book written by Kazuo Inamori, the founder of KYOCERA, a global manufacturer of ceramics and printers, and KDDI, a large Japanese telecommunication enterprise, both FORTUNE 500 companies. More importantly, Inamori has written A *Compass to Fulfillment*, a book on passion and spiritual life in business.

The Japanese perspective presented in Inamori's book paralleled what I believed. The book reinforced the fact that there is a Japanese way of life, a culture of creation, perfection, honesty, and cordial behavior that ultimately helps create harmonious societies, healthy living and beautiful things in life, from food, activities to consumption items.

"Change your thinking and transform your life" is one of many valuable concepts Inamori writes about. This idea perfectly aligns with what I have tried to convey in this book and is one of the main goals of GLUCUT COACHING.

"Your destiny depends on your state of mind" is another truth of his book. When you embark on a path of positive change and start seeing results, you will want to do and achieve more, creating a cycle of lasting success.

Dreams come true when you can visualize every detail. Only when you learn all about pre-diabetes and obesity will you truly control your destiny. Up to that point, you're likely to rely on medicine to solve the problem or ignore it completely until too late . When you embrace this subject as your own, the changes will come naturally, without much effort.

Please don't wait until you are diagnosed with this epidemic health condition. Make a change now!

Hector Hocsman, Osaka Japan, January 2015

1

OVERVIEW

GLUCUT COACHING is a self-paced, lifestyle and behavior modification program based on the healthy lifestyle of the Japanese people. The hallmarks of the program are 500-calorie meals, low stress, moderate physical activity, and balance. You will notice a difference in your appearance and in how you feel, and will develop a positive attitude toward life. The GLUCUT COACHING program is based on my personal experience in Japan, where I found an opportunity to reverse my Diabetes 2 condition and the path I was on, and to live a healthier and more enjoyable life.

If you are **Obese, pre-diabetic or borderline diabetic**, you need to make significant changes to your lifestyle to avoid developing diabetes-related health conditions that can reduce your life expectancy and quality of life. Ignoring your condition beyond the health issue, can have a big affect to your finances and make you dependent on others for care. Embracing the program and lifestyle will create extensive monetary savings to your pocket and community.

The core concept of this program is to empower the individual by reducing dependency on the healthcare system through lowering medications/treatments and food consumption. You'll be able to achieve on average 50% total reduction or more in Medical expenses and Food if you transform your life with this program—all depending on your will power.

When you commit to GLUCUT COACHING, you will experience one of the most amazing periods in your lifetime, an incomparable personal change.

GLUCUT COACHING combines three major components:

1. **GLUCUT COACHING – BOOK** *Theory and Educational material to educate you in the process of personal change (with follow-up tables)*

2. **GLUCUT COACHING – APP** *A Training program App is available for iOS and Android devices. See* www.GLUCUT.com *for instructions*

3. GLUCUT COACHING – PERSONAL COACHING *Assistance to embrace the program*

Both the book and the app will act as the base for your motivational and personal transformation with minimum effort and cost to you. GLUCUT COACHING offers a new approach to lifestyle change based on Japanese culture, which has a proven record of promoting wellness and longevity.

In addition to learning about Japanese culture and lifestyle, possible outcomes include:

- Longevity, extended lifespan
- Reduction in medical expenses
- Reductions in medication dosages
- Fewer medical side effects
- A more positive attitude toward life and yourself
- More physical energy and emotional strength
- Increased stamina
- Lightness
- Awakening – a personal enlightenment
- A deeper relationship with nature
- More energy for work and probable increase in income
- A healthy body and soul
- Lower stress

To achieve these benefits, the program includes the following steps:

1. Initial assessment and evaluation by your healthcare practitioner
2. Diet modification process supervised by a nutritionist
3. Activity modification process coordinated with your Licensed Trainer
4. Emotional modification process coordinated with your spiritual practitioner
5. GLUCUT COACHING – Monitoring your food intake/calorie count, physical activity, body parameters (weight, body fat, visceral

fat, BMI, BMR, TEE, AEE, and others) and elevating your conscious level to better health

6. Introducing examples of healthy living based on the Japanese lifestyle

The GLUCUT COACHING program will help you make healthier lifestyle choices that can potentially fix your condition. It falls under the category of prevention, because if you require the assistance of a doctor, it's usually too late; too much damage has already been done to your body. But diabetes type 2 is reversible to a certain degree depending on your efforts and level of dedication. We have life examples to prove that it is possible to have self control of this condition and those who take matters seriously have completely stopped taking medicine and rely on their new lifestyle.

Because making **changes is difficult to do by yourself**, The GLUCUT COACHING program increases your **consciousness** and **Awareness** and helps you improve your nutrition, activity level, metabolic rate, and achieve your goals with inspiration from the healthy habits of the Japanese lifestyle. We provide the **Dos** and **Don'ts** that are essential for your transformation.

Your condition did not appear overnight. Most likely it developed over years with several contributing factors, such as poor diet, a stressful lifestyle, sedentary behavior, a temperature-controlled environment, limited body perspiration, and other factors with stress being a particularly a key contributor.

When some of the natural processes within your body have been compromised, your body reacts in different ways, often showing some of the following symptoms:

- Overweight
- Fatigue and low energy levels, inability to get out of bed in the morning
- Irregular thirst at all times of day and night
- Urinating at all hours of day (especially at midnight)
- Strong smelling urine (sweet smell) and foamy urine
- Irregular appetite at all times or no appetite

- High and irregular blood sugar (blood glucose) levels with spikes
- High A1C level
- Poor vision—cloudy; sensitivity to daylight
- Skin problems
- Blood not clotting when cut; small bruises
- Nervousness; irritation for no reason
- Depression
- Bad moods and intolerance; disagreeable behavior toward family and close friends
- Internal damage to organs and blood health (can only be monitored by a healthcare provider); damage usually happens after many years and is irreversible.

If you make no lifestyle changes, you are likely to see the condition of your health continue to deteriorate. You will lower your life expectancy and diminish your quality of life, physically, emotionally, and economically.

Actively participating in GLUCUT COACHING will show you how to save tens of thousands of dollars in medical expenses, enjoy a healthier and more pleasant life, and probably extend your life expectancy by many years. With the Average Diabetes 2 bills about $1,000/Month according to CDC (Center of Disease control), reducing the expense by 50% is a significant cumulative change over your lifetime detailed at Chapter D. under Monetary Savings.

As you continue to work with your healthcare provider, we anticipate that over time he or she will reduce your medication as improvement in your condition becomes apparent. Your healthcare provider may even claim this is the result of closely following his medical treatment, but we believe it should be attributed to the natural lifestyle you have embraced.

The GLUCUT COACHING program is based on my personal Lifestyle experience in Japan, where I found an opportunity to change the path I was on, reverse my Type 2 Diabetes and live a healthier life.

Here are the steps I followed:

- **I acknowledged the problem** and figured out what had brought me to that point.

- **I evaluated what I could do to fix the situation** and implemented a new natural lifestyle routine.

- **I considered the current healthcare system** and recognized that I wanted to limit my interactions with the system to routine checkups for as long as I could. I wasn't afraid to ask questions of my practitioner. The more involved I was, the better educated and able to control my actions I became. Once I understood the whole problem, I was motivated by walking, by controlling the quantities of food I consumed, by eating low-fat and quality natural foods, and by having a balanced lifestyle. I began to experience real improvements in my health, without any side effects from medications as I stopped taking them and relied on my healthy new path. I was encouraged to look for alternatives and ultimately to create this lifestyle modification program.

- **I changed habits** (the most difficult thing to do). Better choices became natural and normal, no longer requiring conscious discipline and restraint. Change is a moderate and slow process!

- **I evaluated my overall condition**, monthly at first and later annually, to see how the changes had impacted me physically, emotionally, holistically, and spiritually. I observed changes—both short and long-term, over months and years.

Getting the Most from GLUCUT COACHING

Monitor and track your diet, activities, etc. (See Chapter D. Monitoring for details). The more information you keep track of (daily, weekly, monthly, and yearly), the more you can improve your condition. Use special devices that assist you to see the results, monitor your condition, and take action for change. These include: Fit scale weight, pedometer / calories / activity count, GLUCUT App.

The ultimate goal is to reach a stage where you have achieved a level of **knowledge and practice** and monitoring is not needed any longer with the process done all done unconsciously.

Follow the advice for weekly, monthly, and annual Personal Evaluation Progress Updates emails you will receive as a GLUCUT COACHING participant.

The GLUCUT COACHING program provides self-managed, pre-diabetes support and in no way should be used as a replacement for working with your healthcare provider.

Why COACHING?

Approximately 75% of healthcare costs are related to treating preventable chronic diseases. Take responsibility for your health, and reap the full benefits of optimal health and wellbeing, the foundation for thriving in your personal and professional life.

Professional wellness coaches form partnerships with clients to optimize health and wellbeing by developing and sustaining healthful lifestyles. Coaches help clients increase their level of self-motivation and self-regulation.

Coaches leverage strengths, navigate the journey of change, and build other psychological resources such as mindfulness, optimism, self-efficacy, and resilience, which will help you sustain the changes over time.

Welcome to GLUCUT COACHING!

GLUCUTCOACHING

A
THEORY AND MY STORY

OVERWEIGHT, DIABETES AND HEALTH

Metabolic Syndrome – What is it?

If your blood sugar is high, you might be experiencing common symptoms of diabetes, such as increased thirst and urination, fatigue, and blurred vision. If you have metabolic syndrome or any of the conditions related to metabolic syndrome, **you can delay or even prevent the development of serious health problems by modifying your lifestyle**. GLUCUT COACHING will help you make healthier lifestyle choices.

Often called the "quiet disease" because most of the disorders associated with it show no symptoms until the later stages, **metabolic syndrome** is diagnosed as a cluster of conditions associated with almost irreversible effects.

Conditions, such as **increased blood pressure, high blood sugar levels, excess body fat around the waist, and abnormal cholesterol levels**, typically occur together in Metabolic Syndrome. Any one of these conditions can increase the risks of heart disease, stroke, or diabetes, but when two or more of these conditions occur in combination, your health risk is even greater.

Metabolic syndrome increases the risk of developing cardiovascular disease, particularly heart failure, and diabetes. Some studies have estimated that Diabetes 2, (also called "Type 2") affects more than 9% of the adult population in the US (Center for Disease Control, 2014), and prevalence increases with age. About 32% of the entire population is diagnosed with Obesity/pre-diabetes condition (a level of BMI 30.0 and above) . Overall, 41% of the population (2014) is considered pre-Diabetic or Type 2 Diabetic (CDC).

Type 2 Diabetes - How Did I Get It?

No one who has Type 2 Diabetes really knows exactly when it started and how they got it. In my own case, there were several contributing factors. I led a **sedentary lifestyle** (no activity and minimal sweating) for many years and often ate Restaurant prepared food with high sugar (Sodas of all kind) and sodium (salt) content. I experienced weight gain, especially in the waist area (visceral fat) and a stressful work environment. I had a family history of diabetes and high cholesterol. After 3 or 4 years of having high LDL and low HDL cholesterol, and sugar levels that bordered on high (with many prescription of Statins - cholesterol-lowering-medication which I ignored because of side affects) a doctor informed me I had type 2 diabetes.

My wife and I had been on a wonderful vacation to Italy. There, in the magic city of Venice, I began to feel extremely tired in the mornings, (at 46 years old), staying in bed longer and even letting my wife go on trips in the city by herself, something I would never normally do, especially not in a foreign city. I experienced tremendous **thirst, skin irritation, cloudy vision, dizziness, and unclear thinking**. I felt out of sorts—different enough to make me decide to see a doctor when I returned home.

At first I was in denial. I asked questions like, "How come I feel so unhealthy?" and made statements like, "Nothing is wrong with me or my behavior." Even with high blood sugar readings, I refused to believe I was sick. The fact that I had rarely been sick or taken any medicine in my 46 years was shocking and agitating.

I started a diet right away to lose extra pounds. I began walking every morning, regularly until I began to sweat. I ate healthy portions of the Japanese meals my wife prepared which combine low fat, few calories, small portions, and a variety of vegetables, steamed cooking, and fish.

My blood sugar numbers improved, but were never stable. I had spikes in my blood sugar readings every time I ate different foods, a function the pancreas is supposed to manage.

I came to accept that I did have Type 2 diabetes. With great motivation I sought to reverse the condition. I had to accept that, although I could make healthier choices, my pancreas would never function correctly as before. The pancreas is an endocrine gland that produces several important hormones, including insulin, glucagon, somatostatin, and pancreatic polypeptide which circulate in the blood. The pancreas is also a digestive organ, secreting digestive enzymes that assist digestion and absorption of nutrients in the small intestine. These enzymes help to further break down the carbohydrates, proteins, and lipids in the chyme. Once the pancreas is damaged, the condition cannot be reversed and either you will need to do excessive exercise in order to take no pills insulin or you will need to balance moderate activity with pills for a healthy Glucose readings.

I visited my healthcare provider, a specialist in diabetes, who prescribed different pills. They irritated my stomach, caused pain in my vision, and resulted in thirst—all symptoms I had never experienced before. When I expressed my concerns, all I got was more medical expenses for pills and monitoring devices, but I never felt natural again and felt like I was losing control of my health.

For my 15–30-minute sessions with doctors, I receive 1–2 minutes of orientation on food and exercise and lifestyle changes I needed to make. I never understood the right balance between medicine and lifestyle. This eventually proved to be about half self-controlled lifestyle and half medical monitoring by my healthcare provider in order to achieve a balanced life without symptoms. Eventually I was able to avoid the medicine altogether and rely on monitoring alone.

I started testing my blood sugar before and after meals. I ate different foods in smaller quantities. I slowly began to understand how and what I did and ate affected my condition. Eventually I began working on the GLUCUT COACHING program. I am pleased to offer a simple and easy to read program and guides that help you live a healthier lifestyle and maintain it for the rest of your life.

Today I continue to live the healthy lifestyle described here in this book, knowing that this gives me the best chance to enjoy a long, quality life.

Without GLUCUT COACHING Monitoring

Reliance on the Healthcare System—95%
Dr. Advice for Better Food / Exercise—5%

With GLUCUT COACHING Monitoring

Reliance on the Healthcare System—0 to 50%
Self discipline—Food / Exercise—0 to 50%

Statistics

According to 2014 statistics from the Center for Disease Control, more than 32% of the US population has been diagnosed with a Obesity /pre-diabetes condition. The map opposite shows the spread of the problem and intensity in different US states.

This number represents over a third of the total US population, with an additional 9.2% considered to have type 2 diabetes. The total portion of the US population affected by this disorder is over 41%, a staggering pandemic!

Globally speaking, more than 2 billion people or almost 30% of the global population, are considered overweight or obese. The problem is expected to get worse. Based on current trends, half or (50%) of the world's adults will be overweight or obese by 2030.

According to the University of British Columbia doctors, Pre-Diabetes is a pre-condition, while Type-2 Diabetes is a condition that healthcare insurance companies are devoting major resources to combating. Pre-Diabetes is not considered a disease; therefore many of the related costs are passed to the patient and not covered by insurance companies.

Countries with high GDPs have the highest percentage of Obesity / pre-diabetes and type 2 diabetes cases within their populations. This happens when populations reach higher income levels and increase their use of cars,

Fattest States in USA from 2008 to 2010[1]

climate control (air conditioning), washers and dryers, refrigerators, public transportation, etc. When there are drastic increases in the percentage of Type 2 Diabetes cases, there is generally an increase in the consumption of processed foods. This leads to decreased physical activity, more reliance on motor transportation, and more pollution in the water, air, and soil combined with a stressful lifestyle.

According to the International Diabetes Federation, the greatest increases in numbers of people with diabetes over the next 20 years will occur in low and middle-income countries. The increase is driven by a growing adult population of people who live longer, and by behavior changes associated with rapidly increasing urbanization and development. Key changes in behavior include reduced physical activity (low blood circulation and no sweating), a shift to higher calorie diets, and the associated increases in overweight and obesity. BMI (Body Mass Index) differentiate between Overweight and Obesity. BMI (which is measured by indicating your height and

---

1   (CDC- The Center for Disease Control)

weight) is one of most important and simple indicators for self diagnosis of your health condition. You can Google BMI or find more details in this book.

BMI   **Weight Status**

BMI – BODY MASS INDEX – A formula that measures body fat based on height and weight

BMI Formula: weight (kg) / [height (m)]2

GLUCUTCOACHING **Rule of Thumb**

Calculate your BMI and evaluate your condition.

BMI	Weight Status
Below 18.5	Underweight
18.5 – 24.9	Normal or Healthy Weight
25.0 – 29.9	Overweight
30.0 and Above	Obese

The obesity epidemic has grown too big to ignore. Obesity brings increased cases of disability and premature death, lost productivity, and higher health-care costs. "Obesity, which should be preventable, is now responsible for about 5% of all deaths worldwide." (CNN, 2014). Since being Obese, one can still function, its evident that the balance of Weight vs. Height is in disproportionate levels, and organs specifically the heart is in overdrive mode.

If I tell you to drive your car with overweight you immediately will think about the damage to the engine. So if your body is overloaded above your correct BMI, why not to think your heart (which is our engine) has also a limited capacity to carry before it will completely come to a stop?. This simple comparison analysis should be at the heart of your thoughts!

Example:

My friend has a weight of 240Lb for a body frame of 6'-0" tall. His BMI indicates 32.5 - Obese while the correct weight for this body frame indicates a maximum weight of 180 - 185 Lb = BMI 25.0 for a healthy person. His weight has a total 60 Lb = 25% overloaded. 60 extra Lb over time will definitely do some damage to knees, heart, pancreas, etc. To read more on BMI refer to Center of Disease Control web site: http://www.cdc.gov/healthyweight/assessing/bmi/adult_bmi/index.html#Definition

So what can be done:

On a Micro scale, one should start eating correctly. On the Macro scale among others possibilities are weighty ideas such as redesigning cities (with a dense city core and neighborhoods that encourage walking and bicycling (New Urbanism), and modest ideas like subsidizing healthy meals in schools (Michelle Obama). Both of these changes would generate a good return on the investment.

But fast food giants must play a role too, by changing the menus in their restaurants. This may be easier said than done. Burger King announced in August that it was removing 'Satisfries' from most of its restaurants. These lower-calorie fries had 40% less fat and 30% fewer calories than McDonald's regular fries, but unfortunately they proved less popular than anticipated. Needless to say, the famous American symbol of the hamburger is not going to disappear any time soon. However, what can be changed is our view of **Quantity vs. Quality (QQ)** with respect to food products.

Healthier choices are readily available:
- Eliminate soft drinks from our diets
- Substitute baked potatoes for French fries

- Add a salad as a side order
- Reduce bun size and avoid white flours
- Eat only grass-fed, hormone-free beef and Paltry
- Lower the frequency and quantity of meals
- Eat sustainable wild seafood (Alaskan salmon, cod, trout, halibut, crab, etc.)

All of these choices create a tasty, far healthier meal, without forcing you to suppress your desire for a burger. This is just one aspect of the GLUCUT COACHING approach.

McDonald's has seen tremendous reduction in profitability as new, upgraded burgers chains invade the marketplace. This follows a wave of demand for healthy choices by consumers. It will be the responsibility of the consumer to ultimately change the menu in the marketplace. Your voice is heard any time you shop for better products and that happens only when you are well educated about healthy choices.

GLUCUTCOACHING Action Steps

1. **Get evaluated by a healthcare professional** to determine what condition you have, understand its severity, and get medical advice. Record all data (weight, blood sugar, etc.) in the tables in this book.

2. **Read this book thoroughly** and start with a self-determined program monitoring things you can control, such as food intake and activity level. Read the "food facts" label on each package you consume. Buy organic food, drink mineral water, etc.

3. **Create a Food Program** – Slowly eliminate unhealthy foods described in this book, always in coordination with a nutritionist and healthcare provider.

4. **Create an activity level program.** Start walking. Measure distances and numbers of steps, with the assistance of a pedometer or Smartphone app.

5. **Buy a TANITA Fitscale** (or similar). This will keep you observing major indicators like weight, fat levels, metabolic age, etc. Regularly write down the results in the tables provided in this book.

6. **Evaluate your performance** over weekly, monthly, quarterly, and yearly periods.

7. **Write down and celebrate your improvements**.

8. **Consult with your GLUCUT COACH** periodically to see how he can motivate you further.

9. **Download the GLUCUT APP** when available for better results.

HEALTH and LIFESTYLE

It will shock no one to hear that Americans are remarkably unhealthy eaters.

Guardian Newspaper

Introduction

America and the western world is experiencing a wave of natural and healthy lifestyle change. It started with movements introduced in California during the 1970s with famous people like Jane Fonda, and other Hollywood persona advocating aerobics, yoga and natural, healthy foods.

The health revolution seems to follow wealth and economic progress. It is associated with and embraced by people within the higher echelon of wealth and consumption. The computer revolution opened the awareness to the middle classes.

Today, new chains offering grass-fed beef hamburgers are appearing like mushrooms after the rain, and endangering giants such as McDonalds and Burger King with alternative healthier products.

GLUCUT COACHING will help you become part of this revolution. Though lifestyle change doesn't happen overnight, you will find that alternative natural foods taste great, increase your energy level, and decrease the harmful fats and sugars that have been damaging your body.

Food Consumption - Modifying your Diet

A new American Diet Report Card confirms that we eat too much cheese, sugar, starch, and red meat and not enough fruits and vegetables. We consume 500 more calories per day on average than we did in the 1970s. An average intake of 2,640 calories for men and 1,785 calories per day for women has been recorded by the USDA (2014).

Important Note: This program recommends closely monitoring your diet; consult with a licensed dietitian or nutritionist to establish how many calories you should eat every day.

> Limiting the amount of food you eat is an important component of a Healthy Diet
>
> **Energy IN = Energy OUT**

GLUCUTCOACHING **Rule of Thumb**

1. **Use a smaller plate**; this change will cause you to eat less.

2. In restaurants, **cut your serving in half** and take the rest home. Ask for a doggie bag when you order so you can divide the serving before you start eating. Order appetizers instead of full meals.

3. **Eat 70–80% of your stomach's capacity.**

4. **Eat with a schedule in mind**—3 balanced meals per day.

Healthy Foods
- Vegetables
- Fruits

- Fish and sustainable food of all kinds
- Nuts (moderate amounts)
- Low-fat organic, and grass fed meats
- Boil or Sauté food vs. frying in fat or oil

Unhealthy Foods

- Sodas—contain lots of sugar (colas, artificial sweeteners, juices, etc.) There are 7 spoons of sugar in each can of soda!
- Carbohydrates—pasta, white rice, potatoes, breads, white flour, and alcohol
- Pizza—contains saturated fat from cheese
- Burgers—avoid processed red meat (most fast-food hamburgers are less than 15% beef)
- Fried food—saturated fat/grease/cholesterol

The following formula summarizes the number of calories a person needs to consume daily in order to have a balanced Diet.

> BMR X Activity Levels

BMR = Basal Metabolic Rate—the number of calories needed to sustain a body without any activity.

Activity Level—the activity level of a person affects the number of calories consumed. Values vary from:

- Sedentary—1.2
- Moderate Activity—1.35
- Active in the Gym 4 times per week—1.55
- Very active day labor—1.7

A 2,000-calorie-per-day diet should contain less than 66 grams of fat, less than 20 grams of saturated fat, less than 2,400 milligrams of sodium, and less than 300 grams of total carbohydrate, including sugars. These numbers will vary based on the **Basal Metabolic Rate** (BMR X Activity level) of each individual person.

As no one can continuously monitor the intake of fat, sodium, carbohydrates, etc., GLUCUT COACHING will help make you intuitively conscious of the calorie counts and other aspects of the foods you eat and by doing so you have created awareness.

Calories = Energy—A calorie is simply a unit of energy the body gets from food. The body needs this energy to function just like a car needs gasoline to run. Every person needs a different number of calories each day. The number of calories you need depends on numerous factors, such as:

- Gender
- Age
- Weight
- Height
- Activity level

Cut excess calories from your diet to the level your body needs to function. Moderation is the key element in diet. Use an online Calorie Calculator such as (www.mayoclinic/calorie-calculator).

Once you start reducing your caloric intake, you will likely experience hunger at first; it takes 1-3 years for your stomach to adjust to a balanced caloric intake. "Balanced" means you eat the same number of calories each day that your body consumes for fuel. It can take months to reduce your body's excess fat. Reducing stomach size and psychological desire takes years. The moment of truth comes when your forbidden favorite food is laid in front of you and you have no desire to eat it.

Dieting and lifestyle change are difficult for the same reasons that unhealthy eating is easy. If you eat a piece of cake with ice cream, the excess fat won't show up on your stomach the next week or even the next month. Becoming obese and unhealthy is a gradual, cumulative process where we are fooled into thinking that the cake has "disappeared" when we step on a scale the next day. When we forego the piece of cake and skip dessert, that act of discipline does not bring about a direct, noticeable result. Becoming healthy is also a gradual, cumulative process and unfortunately, a piece of cake delivers a lot more instant gratification than an empty plate. Plenty of diets promise quick rewards, which is why most of them fail. The rewards of GLUCUT COACHING are real, but don't get discouraged if 2–3 months of discipline doesn't look or feel like much. **Lifestyle changes are lifetime commitments**. Stick with the guidelines offered here and you'll feel good, look good, and have much to be proud of.

When I moved to Japan, I often experienced a need to eat immediately after a meal as the portions served are about half what we eat in the USA. Slowly, I reduced the quantities of food in my meals to a point where my stomach and energy levels adjusted to the new me. Years passed. My BMI (Body Mass Index) is in the healthy levels, and I am conscious of what I consume, actively and naturally keeping myself healthy.

GLUCUTCOACHING **Rule of Thumb**

> Eat Breakfast Like a King, Lunch like a Prince,
> and Dinner like a Poor man

BREAKFAST

Breakfast truly is the most important meal of the day. Our bodies rely on energy to move in the morning after starving during the night. A breakfast of 400–500 calories is a good target for achieving weight loss and wellbeing. A serving of oatmeal is about 68 calories per 100 grams, fruits are 53 calories per 100 grams, and nuts are 576 calories per 100 grams. Try to balance the meal: 68 +53 + 192 (576/3) = 313 calories. Add a slice of toast with low-fat margarine or olive oil to make 100 calories. That's 413 calories for breakfast. After I adjusted my diet, this breakfast satisfied me, but it took a year of hunger and repeated breakfast modifications before I made a full adjustment.

Three samples of 400–600 Calorie Breakfasts:

- The most recommended breakfast is OATMEAL (with added fruits and nuts). OATMEAL (especially whole or steel-cut oats) is high in fiber, low in calories, fulfilling, easy to digest, and will carry you from early morning to early afternoon, an excellent way to lose weight and keep energy levels up. You can also go for a salty hot meal with miso soup and vegetables.

- 1 egg, 1 slice of toast with low-fat margarine or one slice of cheese, coffee and milk with 1 tsp. brown sugar, a small salad, a small yogurt (You will feel hungry 2 hours after eating.)

- Fruits, vegetable salad (You will feel hungry 2 hours after eating.)

LUNCH

Timing is important at lunch. Keep a fixed schedule between 1–2PM. Eat moderately and do not avoid this meal. Try to eat about 500–600 calories for lunch.

Sample meal:

- 100 grams of meat, small portion of baked potato, salad, ice/hot tea
- Mixed salad with grilled chicken
- Wrap with avocado, salad and meat/chicken

Dinner

Timing of dinner is also important. Have a fixed schedule during evenings, too. Do not eat after 7 PM. You should eat about 500 calories at dinner.

Sample meal:

- 100 grams of fresh fish, a small portion of miso soup, salad, iced/hot tea

Total per day—1500 calories + 200-calorie morning snack + 200-calorie afternoon snack = 1,900 Calories (Correct for a 164Lb , 5'-7"Male Diet)

GLUCUTCOACHING Rule of Thumb

> Do not eat at night. Eat before 7PM.

Healthy Eating Behaviors

- **Eat 70–80% of your stomach's capacity**—allow room for stomach activity
- **Monitor IQ**—Intake Quantities control—Balance the intake of calories to match the amount of calories consumed by your body. Use the Tanita AM 120E monitor or a like to measure TEE (Total Energy Expenditure), which means the total number of calories you consume per day (including activity, sleeping, and resting)
- **Reduce Portions**—Keep around 500 calories per meal
- **Do not eat after 7 PM**—Allow time for food to digest before going to bed
- **Fried Food**— Avoid completely
- **Sodas**—Avoid completely, including all artificial, sugary juices
- **Don't drink while eating**—Avoid drinking during meals to allow better digestion
- **Drink water**—Drink lots of natural spring water during the day to

cleanse your body and lower sugar levels between meals. Avoid tap or purified water.

- **Avoid carbohydrates** (rice, bread, potatoes, pasta)—Eat carbohydrates in moderation, never at evening meals

- **Eat organic food** as much as possible

- **Eat fruits and vegetables** as much as possible

- **Dairy**—Avoid or eat moderately

- **Reduce animal protein/meats**—Keep to 100 gram per meals (chicken, pork, red meat, fish)

- **Reduce Stress**—Avoid news and bad habits. Rest moderately. Enjoy good company and reading. Go outdoors and engage in physical activities.

- **Eat only when you're hungry** – Avoid recreational eating

- **Walk daily until you sweat**, especially after eating to help digestion. Doctors suggest a minimum of 10,000 steps each day, an equivalent of 30 minutes of walking at 3 miles per hour.

- **Indulge yourself**—Start by allowing yourself to eat favorite forbidden foods you crave such as pizza, burgers, French fries, sweets, etc. foods twice each month. Slowly cut back to one time per month just to get a taste and a lasting feeling. Your body will eventually tell you don't need them anymore.

METABOLIC RATE

Metabolic Syndrome is a condition where the body slows down its function. To enhance the metabolic rate, eat less, feel hunger without responding to it instantly, sweat, move your body, sun bathe (with proper sunscreen), shower and cleanse your body (massaging every part of it slowly and deeply), listen to yourself (body and mind), be in touch with nature, breathe clean air (at the beach/sea level), reduce stress, be socially positive, be happy and live with compassion.

Unhealthy Behaviors — Things to Avoid

- Avoid eating processed food instead of natural or organic options
- Avoid eating more calories than you burn
- Avoid eating at the wrong hours (eating late at night)
- Avoid eating poor food combinations
- Avoid eating excessive sugar
- Avoid living an inactive lifestyle
- Avoid drinking too much alcohol
- Avoid not exercising/sedentary living
- Avoid smoking or using drugs
- Avoid not sweating; having a slow metabolic rate
- Avoid living in wrong room temperatures (A/C with constant, monitored temperature) (shutting down the natural sweating system in our bodies)
- Avoid fast eating; swallowing before chewing thoroughly
- Avoid drinking during meals
- Avoid not drinking enough water during the day (spring mineral water recommended)
- Avoid little or no exposure to nature - sun, wind, and more
- Avoid red meats
- Avoid fried foods
- Avoid sodas and high content sugar drinks
- Avoid carbohydrates (breads, rice, pasta, starch/potatoes) — South Beach Diet
- Do not eat after 7PM — This allows the body to digest and burn food before you go to sleep
- Moderate alcohol intake
- Avoid high-calorie sweets — cakes, cookies
- Avoid highly processed foods

The Food Movement[1]

We usually take food for granted. The history of food consumption from the stone age forward goes from hunting to agrarian societies and to the modern age of urban settlement.

By abandoning the agrarian life, we embarked on a much easier but less healthy path. Once, people of the islands consumed primarily natural fish, while inland people consumed primarily grass-fed beef. Today, this order is non-existent, with sushi bars offering farmed fish, and meat treated with hormones and antibiotics. We feed our bodies with diets that are strangers to our evolution. We have changed our diet more in the past 50 years than during the entire preceding millennium.

Two primary changes are significant: First, we have stopped the body activity associated with farming. Two: we started consuming processed foods combined with overeating. **Physical activity and healthy consumption are essential to a balanced metabolic rate**.

Americans spend a smaller percentage of their income on food than any people in history—slightly less than 10 percent—and a smaller amount of time preparing it: a mere thirty-one minutes per day on average, including cleanup.

The US Food and Drug Administration's cheap food policy worked almost too well. Crop prices fell, forcing farmers to produce more to simply break even. This led to a deep depression in the farm belt during the 1980s followed by a brutal wave of consolidation. Most importantly, the price of food came down, or at least the price foods that could be made from corn and soy: processed foods and sweetened beverages and feedlot meat.

The Food Movement's strongest claim getting public attention today is that the American diet of highly processed food laced with added fats and sugars is responsible for the epidemic of chronic diseases that threatens to bankrupt the healthcare system. The Center for Disease Control estimates that fully three quarters of US health care spending goes to treat chronic

---

1   http://www.nybooks.com/articles/archives/2010/jun/10/food-movement-rising/

diseases, most of which are preventable and linked to diet: heart disease, stroke, type 2 diabetes, and at least a third of all cancers. The health care crisis probably cannot be addressed without addressing the catastrophe of the American diet, and that diet is the direct (if unintended) result of the way that our agriculture and food industries have been organized.

GLUCUT COACHING advocates a reverse process. Eat natural non-processed foods in low quantities, and enhance your day with routine physical activities as much you can.

CALORIES IN FOOD

Nutrition Facts (sample)

100 gram Hamburger Patty	100 gram Pizza	100 gram Salad
295 calories	265 calories	17 calories

The average person consumes 300–400 grams of food in each meal. The foods listed above, except salad, all surpass the average meal in caloric content (500 Calories meals we advocate). Meals that come with breads, mayonnaise, and sauce can easily reach more than 1,000 calories. In the table above, a 300-gram pizza is over 795 calories, and that's without the drink and dessert. This example amplifies the problem that one can't notice the quantity of calories consumed unless you research it. **This pizza and hamburgers meals surpasses 1,000 calories!**

Research the portions and calorie counts of the foods you need to be eating.

GLUCUT—Modification Method: A thin crust 14-inch pizza has 192 calories / slice x 2 slices = 384 calories. Add dessert and a drink and you can achieve the 500—600 calorie per meal goal. That will satisfy a craving for pizza once a month.

TEE - Calculating Total Energy Expenditure

One of the easiest and most effective methods of managing food intake is to calculate your daily **TEE = Total Energy Expenditure**: The number of calories you need to eat each day on average in order to maintain your current body weight.

Set a daily calorie target based on your TEE to lose weight at the healthy rate of ½ to −1 pound a week. Fat accumulates in our body slowly over time. Any adjustment in the opposite direction will show results slowly, but steadily.

Most anyone will lose weight on a daily diet of 1,500 calories. Nutritionists do not recommend daily calorie goals of less than 1,200 because at that level it's hard to meet your nutritional needs or to feel satisfied enough to stick to a plan.

I. Alternative Method for calculating your TEE

> TEE: Your Current Weight (Lb) x 12 = daily calories to maintain current weight

Example:

If you weigh 165 pounds, multiply 165 X 12 to find that you can maintain your weight by eating 1,900 calories a day.

- **To lose 1 pound each week**, cut 500 calories a day.
- **To lose 2 pounds each week**, cut 1,000 calories a day.

An example of a 1,900 calorie a day diet based on GLUCUT COACHING: 500 calories x 3 meals each day = 1500 calories + 200 calorie snack + 200 calorie snack.

IMPORTANT NOTE: Always talk with your healthcare provider or a nutritionist before making changes to your diet.

2. Alternative Method for calculating your TEE

You can also identify your TEE by multiplying your Basal Metabolic Rate by your Activity level.

> TEE—Total Energy Expenditure
> = Current weight (lbs.) x 12
> = BMR X Activity Level

First, calculate your BMR using the **Mifflin-St. Jeor** equation where:

(w = weight (kg), h = height (cm), y = years/age)

> BMR Women: (9.99 x w) + (6.25 x h) – (4.92 x y) – 161
> BMR Men: (9.99 x w) + (6.25 x h) – (4.92 x y) + 5

Next, identify your Activity level.

- **Sedentary**: $1.0 - 1.3$ (Average 1.2)
- **Mild / Low Active**: $1.3 - 1.5$ (Average 1.35)
- **Medium Active**: $1.5 - 1.6$ (Average 1.55)
- **Moderate Active**: $1.6 - 1.85$ (Average 1.725)
- **Extreme Active**: $1.85 - 2.0$ (Average 1.9)

If you are a 55-year-old male who is 5'-7" tall and - weighs 164 pounds, your BMR would be 1,626.

BMR: (9.99 x w) + (6.25 x h) – (4.92 x y) + 5
TEE = BMR x Activity Level = Weight (lb) X 12

TEE = 1,626 x 1.2 sedentary = 1,951 calories a day:

- 500 Calories Breakfast
- 550 Calories Lunch
- 500 Calories Dinner
- Snacks – Coffee, Cookie – 200 calories x 2 = 400 calories

Total = 1,950 calories a day in order to maintain weight. Eating fewer than 1,950 calories a day will slowly decrease fat tissue. (TEE – Total calories needed depends on the Activity Factor). http://www.bmi-calculator. net/bmr-calculator/

ACTIVITY LEVELS FACTORS EXPLANATION—HARRIS BENEDICT FACTOR

The Harris Benedict Equation is a formula that uses your BMR and then applies an activity factor to determine your total daily energy expenditure (calories). The only factor omitted by the Harris Benedict Equation is lean body mass. Remember, leaner bodies need more calories than less leaner ones. Therefore, this equation will be very accurate in all but the very muscular (will underestimate calorie needs) and the very fat (will overestimate calorie needs).

Activity Levels Index

- **Sedentary**: Little to no regular exercise. Office worker with no activity (Factor 1.2)

- **Mild activity level**: Intensive exercise for at least 20 minutes 1–3 times per week. This may include bicycling, jogging, basketball, swimming, skating, etc. If you do not exercise regularly, but you maintain a busy life style that requires you to walk frequently for long periods, you meet the requirements of this level. (Factor 1.375)

- **Moderate activity level**: Intensive exercise for at least 30 to 60 minutes 3–4 times per week. Any of the activities listed above will qualify. (Factor 1.55)

- **Heavy or (Labor-intensive) activity level**: Intensive exercise for 60 minutes or greater 5–7 days per week (see sample activities above). Labor-intensive occupations also qualify for this level. Labor-intensive construction work (brick laying, carpentry, general labor, farming, landscaping, etc.) (Factor 1.7)

- **Extreme level**: Exceedingly active and/or very demanding activities: Examples: (1) athlete with an almost unstoppable training schedule with multiple training sessions throughout the day (2) very demanding job, such as shoveling coal or working long hours on an assembly line. Generally, this level of activity is very difficult to achieve. (Factor 1.9)

METs - Activity Intensity

The Metabolic Equivalent of Task (MET) is a physiological measure that expresses the energy costs of physical activities. Though a formula is explained below, you don't have to understand it or perform any calculations yourself). The Tanita Activity Monitor (discussed on page 35) does the work for you, and MET values offer a simple and convenient way to monitor and track how much energy you're burning.

Actual energy expenditure (e.g., in calories or joules) during an activity depends on a person's body mass. The energy cost of a given activity will be different for persons of different weights. MET is used as a means of expressing comparable intensity and energy expenditure between persons of different weight.

MET is defined as the ratio of metabolic rate (and therefore the rate of energy consumption) during a specific physical activity to a referenced metabolic rate, set by convention to 3.5 ml $O2 \cdot kg^{-1} \cdot min^{-1}$ or equivalently.

There are three MAIN distinct INTENSITY LEVELS of activity:

$$1 \text{ MET} \equiv 1\frac{\text{kcal}}{\text{kg} * h} \equiv 4.184\frac{\text{kJ}}{\text{kg} * h}$$

1. Sedentary activity+ (RED)
   0.9 -1.0 METs* Sleeping / Sitting at rest
2. Low/Moderate activity+ (BLUE)
   2.0 to 6.0 METs* (3.5 to 7 calories/min) – Fast Walking (3-5 Km/H)
3. Vigorous activity+ (GREEN)
   Greater than 6.0-10 METs* (more than 7 calories/min) – Jogging / Push Ups

MET is an index of the intensity of activities. For example, an activity with a MET value of 2, such as walking at a slow pace (e.g. 3 km/h) would require twice the energy that an average person consumes at rest MET value 1 (e.g. sitting quietly).

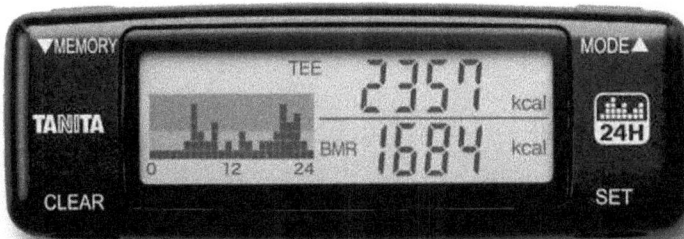

The **Tanita Activity Monitor /Pacer's** measurements are based on inputting your weight, height, and age. It measures walking and running activity and displays BMR, TEE, AEE, number of steps, time spent walking, and METs.

The core reason to use such a device is **motivation**. It reminds you how many calories you should consume each day, and the total calories you burn by walking. (If you run or swim, this device won't measure those results.

Rely on other methods such as researching how many calories the average person burns in an hour of activity).

The TANITA AM120E displays your Activity intensity levels. Each square equals 1 MET. The lower horizontal line shows the level at rest. The line between the blue and brown is about 3.5 METs where you feel intensity levels and initiation of sweat. By displaying your activity results immediately, this monitor encourages you to be active.

Important Note: Always talk with your healthcare provider when looking for activities that best suit your condition.

Detoxification (weekly, monthly, annually)

Our bodies naturally detoxify themselves every day as part of their normal process, eliminating pollutants we absorb from the air and water. Eliminating and neutralizing toxins through the colon, liver, kidneys, lungs, and skin is one of the body's most basic functions.

Bodily systems and organs that were once naturally capable of cleaning out unwanted substances are now completely overloaded to the point where toxic materials remain in our tissues. Contemporary diets, which often include too much animal protein, saturated and trans-fats, caffeine, and alcohol, radically alter our internal biology. Our bodies protect us from dangerous substances by isolating and surrounding the substances with mucous and fat so they will not cause an imbalance or trigger an immune response (Some people carry up to 15 extra pounds of mucous that harbors this waste. The TANITA BC 585 Fit scale, or a similar professional scale, can measure this VISCERAL FAT).

What is the benefit of using a sophisticated Scale? – It helps you acknowledge your body's true condition. Reading that your metabolic age is 44 when you are 55 years old, is a great motivator for maintaining your diet. The same is true when basal rate and body fat levels are in line with healthy standards. A traditional scale measures only weight. A lifestyle scale

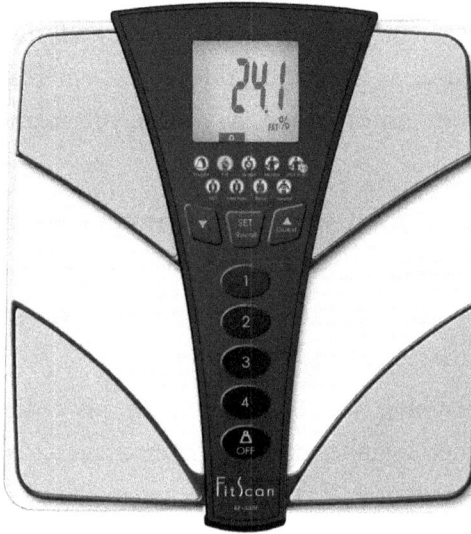

TANITA BC 585 – Fit Scale (Example for a comprehensive scale)

knows a few things about your height, body type, and other factors. It considers your weight as one variable that affects many others, and is therefore able to provide more useful information and lifestyle monitoring.

Monitoring is a GLUCUT COACHING Technique

Cleansing a Healthy Diet

The Story of the Human Body: Evolution, Health and Disease by D. Lieberman explains the evolutionary changes in our diet over the past 10,000 years.

Special cleansing diets are the best way to assist your body's natural self-cleaning system. For those with immune system-compromising diseases like cancer, arthritis, diabetes, and chronic fatigue, detoxification is especially important.

GLUCUT COACHING helps you cleanse your body by promoting a healthier diet, exercise, and emotional stability, all through moderation without being excessive. Over time, this process will make you feel better about yourself, your priorities, and the choices you are making.

EMPLOYERS ARE MEASURING WORKERS' WAISTLINES

Employers want trimmer workers. Weight is the main concern for many employers since so many Americans are too heavy. Nearly 7 in 10 adults are overweight, and more than one-third are obese.

Companies are going beyond just handing out pedometers and offering Weight Watchers memberships. The latest trend is to offer rewards (and penalties) for those who are at risk, in order to make them take action.

Wellness programs have been around for years, but they are evolving. Some companies are performing more biometric screenings. They measure waist circumferences, cholesterol, blood sugar levels, and blood pressure, using independent third-party vendors to protect confidential employee data.

The competition for jobs is increasing exponentially in the past decade as computers and economic trends are changing the workforce. This trend involved more scrutiny in appearance but also in the health of workers as companies are expecting more productivity and want to limit the exposure to absentee workers which is directly related their health.

Sweating and Activities
(Walking, Bicycling, Steps, Gym, Swimming)

Maintaining a moderate level of activity is vital to keeping a healthy balanced lifestyle. **Evaporative heat loss** is critical for human survival in a hot environment, particularly when environmental temperature is higher than skin temperature. Exercise or exposure to a hot environment elevates internal and skin temperatures, and subsequently increases sweat rate and blood flow to the skin.

It is my personal belief that the body requires cleansing through sweating. Modern life deprives the body of this natural phenomenon, and it's showing up as a type 2 diabetes symptom with a high level of sweating as the body tries to clean itself and reduce heat loads.

When going about your regular daily activities, try to be active until your body sweats when possible. Sweating on a regular basis as a result of physical activity increases blood circulation and subsequently lowers sugar levels significantly.

Even light to moderate exercise can make a difference. A leisurely stroll after a meal provides a dramatic drop in dangerously high levels of blood sugar.

Calorie-Burning Chart

Calorie-Burning Chart for Various Activities
Approximate calories burned, per hour, by a 150-pound woman

Exercise	Calories/hour	Exercise	Calories/hour
Sleeping	55	Water Aerobics	400+
Eating	85	Skating/blading	420+
Sewing	85	Dancing, aerobic	420+
Knitting	85	Aerobics	450+
Sitting	85	Bicycling, moderate	450+
Standing	100	Jogging, 5mph	500+
Driving	110	Gardening, digging	500+
Office Work	140	Swimming, active	500+
Housework, moderate	60+	Cross country ski machine	500+
Golf, with trolley	180	Hiking	500+
Golf, without trolley	240	Step Aerobics	550+
Gardening, planting	250	Rowing	550+
Dancing, ballroom	260	Power Walking	600+
Walking, 3mph	280+	Cycling, studio	650
Table Tennis	290+	Squash	650+
Gardening, hoeing etc.	350+	Skipping with rope	700+
Tennis	350+	Running	700+

Use this chart to figure out how many calories you burn through physical activity. Men should add 10% to the number of calories burned per hour as the table is based on women's activities. Table taken from Wikipedia.

GLUCUTCOACHING **Rule of Thumb**

Look for Opportunities to Become More Physically Active

- **Avoid driving** when possible. Walk to the bus, train, or subway

- **Walk up and down stairs** when you can. Avoid elevators

- **Carry your shopping bags** when shopping instead of using a shopping cart, park at the edge of the parking lot to walk longer distances

- **Carry a backpack to work**—a daily activity you will not even notice

- **Go for walks after dinners**

- **Use the TANITA Activity Level Monitor** – monitoring will keep you aware of your daily activity level

All of these regular activities will contribute to your health without requiring you to visit a gym. The effects of small exercises built into your daily routine are cumulative. Walk a half-mile to and from work and you'll add 5 miles of weekly walking to your lifestyle.

Those routines become part of your new activity level without requiring major change to your daily life. By cardio-exercising for longer periods at low and medium intensity, you will achieve more results than by going to the gym and loading your body with high intensity exercise over short periods.

Less Obvious Results of Exercise

You will enjoy physical and emotional benefits when you raise your activity level.

- More efficient use of your body's insulin resulting in lower blood sugar levels

- Reduced amounts of medication needed to control your condition

- Removal of toxins from the body through sweating
- Burning of extra body fat (overall fat and visceral fat)
- Strengthening of muscle tissue and bones
- Reduced blood pressure and improved circulation
- Decreased LDL ("bad") cholesterol
- Increased HDL ("good") cholesterol
- Reduced chances of heart disease and stroke
- Boosted energy and mood (resulting in better sex life)
- Lowered stress and enhanced wellbeing, resulting in better personal relationships
- Improved mood —you'll feel happier than you were before entering the program

GLUCUTCOACHING Action Step

Read this chapter again 3 times until it becomes an integral part of your routine.

Ways to Burn 200 Calories

Do jumping jacks for 2.5 minutes (break into intervals of 30 seconds or one minute)

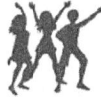

Have a 37 minute dance party

Have a 40 minute game of badminton

An hour of pitch and putt

Do 40 minutes of garden work (25 minutes of uprooting weeds and 15 minutes of planting new seedlings)

An hour of bowling

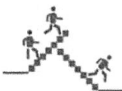

Run up and down the stairs for 2.5 minutes

Wash and wax your car for 40 minutes

PHYSICAL HEALTH, MENTAL HEALTH, and MOTIVATION

Life Expectancy and Quality of Life

Not only is **life expectancy** a prime consideration, **quality of life** is important, too. How long will you be able to stay independent? To walk without assistance? To live without taking medication? How long will you enjoy clear vision, the joy of a sex life, and all the other daily activities you currently take for granted?

According to a December 6, 2014 BBC report, being severely obese can knock up to eight years off your life and cause decades of ill health. A team at McGill University in Canada found that heart problems and type 2 diabetes were major sources of disability and death.

A recent report in The Lancet Diabetes and Endocrinology used computer modeling to calculate the impact of weight on life expectancy. Compared to overweight 20 to 39-year-olds, severely obese men of the same age lost 8.4 years of life. Women lost 6.1 years on average.

Men also spent 18.8 more years living in poor health, while women lived for 19.1 years in that state. For those in their forties and fifties, men lost 3.7 years and women 5.3 years to obesity. Those in their sixties and seventies lost one year of life due to obesity, but still faced 7 years of poor health. Consider the discomfort, medical expense, and even the cumulative costs of harmful, unhealthy, and unnecessary food over 7 years.

Mental Health

There is a straight-line correlation between physical and mental health. Here are common reactions from people upon being diagnosed with diabetes:

- **Anger** - Diabetes is the perfect breeding ground for anger.

- **Denial** - Denial is that voice inside that repeats, "Not me." Most people go through this when first diagnosed.

- **Depression** - Studies show that people with diabetes have a greater risk of depression than people without diabetes.

- **Aggression** - Levels of aggression can increase and damage personal relationships.

See more at: http://www.diabetes.org/living-with-diabetes/complications/mental-health/#sthash.cIlNFdm0.dpuf

Stress Disorder

Stress results when something causes your body to behave as if it were under attack. Sources of stress can be physical, like injury or illness, or they can be mental, like problems with your marriage, job, health, or finances.

When stress occurs, the body prepares to take action. This preparation is called the **fight-or-flight response**. Levels of many hormones shoot up. Their net effect is to make a lot of stored energy—glucose and fat—available to cells. These cells are then primed to help the body get away from danger. In people who have diabetes, the fight-or-flight response does not work well. Insulin is not always able to let extra energy into the cells, so glucose piles up in the blood. High blood sugar results in increased anxiety and a decrease in ability to think rationally and calmly.

I encountered real life examples of people who went through extreme stress and ended with Diabetes Type 2 condition as a result of economic hardship, work related, personal relations , etc. Although this may be also related to other conditions, there is no doubt that stress is a key component.

Diabetic Neuropathies

Diabetic neuropathies are a family of nerve disorders caused by diabetes. People with diabetes can, over time, develop nerve damage throughout the body. Some people with nerve damage have no symptoms. Others experience pain, tingling, or numbness—loss of feeling—in the hands, arms, feet, and legs. Nerve problems can occur in every organ system, including the digestive tract, heart, and sex organs. Common signs of neuropathy are loss of sensation in toes and fingertips, impaired vision and dysfunction in sex.

About 60 to 70 percent of people with diabetes experience some form of neuropathy. People with diabetes can develop nerve problems at any time, but risk increases with age and duration of diabetes. The highest rates of neuropathy are among people who have had diabetes for at least 25 years. Diabetic neuropathies are more common in people who have problems controlling their blood sugar, as well as in those with high levels of blood fat, high blood pressure, and overweight.

The most common symptoms of diabetic neuropathy include stress, edginess, intolerance, palpitations, antisocial behavior, seclusion, and animosity.

Impact on Emotional Health and Sex Life

Emotional wellbeing and sexual activity decrease with obesity. You can reverse this situation by bringing your **BMI (Body Mass Index)** in line with your age, height, and weight.

For men, diabetes can cause damage to the nervous system over a sustained period of time, also known as diabetic neuropathy. One aspect of this is the potential for diabetes to damage the erectile tissue leaving it impossible for a man to achieve or maintain an erection.

Almost 1 in 3 men with diabetes suffer from erectile dysfunction.

Erectile dysfunction can be the way in which men discover that they have diabetes.

However, through strict management of the disease through diet, exercise, pills and insulin injections, minor sexual problems usually recede and it is possible for the man to achieve and erection.

Motivation

Significant lifestyle changes cannot be accomplished without motivation. Acceptance of your condition and the desire to live a healthier life will help you take positive actions and maintain healthier choices.

No matter your stage or condition, **small, manageable, sustainable changes** are the best route forward to reduce your risk of heart disease, impotence, blindness, and other pre-diabetes and type 2 diabetes complications to live a happier, healthier, and longer life. Most diets and exercise routines fail because the patient attempts an "extreme makeover." Introduce small lifestyle changes slowly and deliberately. Allow yourself time to become comfortable with one change before attempting another.

BEHAVIOR MODIFICATION

What Is It?

GLUCUT COACHING is an all-natural, medication-free, self-paced, **lifestyle/behavior modification** experience where you will replace bad habits with healthy behaviors and make them into lasting changes. Behavior modification uses techniques such as altering one's behaviors and reactions to stimuli through positive and negative reinforcement. Behavior modification is a process that occurs over time.

The Process (The Goal, Stepping Stones, and Rewards)

The Goal is clear: a reduction in blood sugar and fat levels, a reduction in medicine, and better health with overall cost savings.

Stepping Stones (small steps) are the healthiest way to modify behavior. Daily reinforcements are the most effective.

Follow a daily routine, from blood testing, to food intake, to activity/exercise and self-consciousness. Inputting your pacer (pedometer) data into GLUCUT COACHING will provide continuous tracking and monitoring of your progress in the program, and will establish patterns of behavior and consciousness that are crucial to success.

The process of imputing data is stressful and with time, once you have engaged in the behavior change, there is no more need for data management. Therefore, data management is a temporary instrument to achieve a lasting behavior change.

Rewards come in the form of feeling healthier and more self-confident. A "forbidden meal" once in a while is an acceptable way to reduce the feelings of guilt one may experience from time to time as a result of eating unhealthy foods that were once part of your daily lifestyle. Eat these foods infrequently as "rewards" for continuous "good behavior." As you progress in the program and begin to feel better, your sense of wellbeing and accomplishment will supersede your desire to claim these rewards.

Used originally by sports and physical fitness enthusiasts, **pedometers** are now becoming popular as everyday exercise measurers and lifestyle motivators. A pacer/pedometer is a device, usually portable and electronic or electromechanical, that counts each step a person takes by detecting the mo-

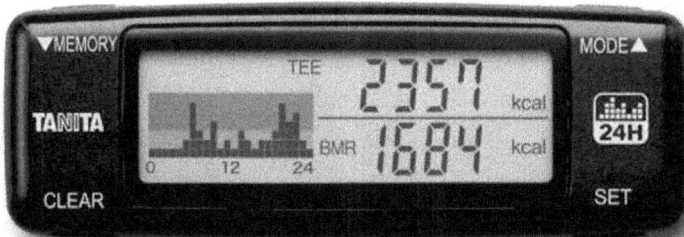

Tanita Monitoring Devise Measure—BMR, TEE, AEE, STEPS, TIME, ACTIVITY LEVEL

tion of the person's hips. Because the distance of each person's step varies, an informal calibration, performed by the user, is required if accurate calculation of the distance covered is desired. New pedometers use electronics and software to automatically determine how a person's step varies by using GPS technology. The Apple iPhone comes with a built in App that measures few of those parameters.

Way of Thinking - Positive vs. Negative

Your self-esteem is important. Pre-diabetes is a condition, not a disease. It revolutionized my life because as a result of the way I responded to my condition, I feel better, eat healthier, have more balanced energy levels, enjoy things in different ways, and appreciate life more than before. Look positive into the future and engage in positive thinking knowing that the condition is reversible. Those who will give up in the process, will confront the unfortunate doors of hospitals and doctors.

The Three-Way Theory

When tracking your results, divide **food, activity, and motivation** into three levels: (small/red = bad, moderate/yellow = borderline, and high/green= good).

Everyday changes are small and harder to notice; such changes do not usually provide motivation. Take small steps. Feel the results. Numbers don't tell the average person anything; stepping-stone results do. If you see your monitored weight change over 1, 2, 3, months, you will see visible results.

The same is true for exercise. One can appreciate climbing stairs without breathing heavily, or strengthening the legs muscles after large walks, and enjoying an improvement in sex life after long periods of low stamina. All these results are within the grasp of the average person. Use them to motivate yourself. The more you change, the more motivated you will be to continue to change and achieve your goals.

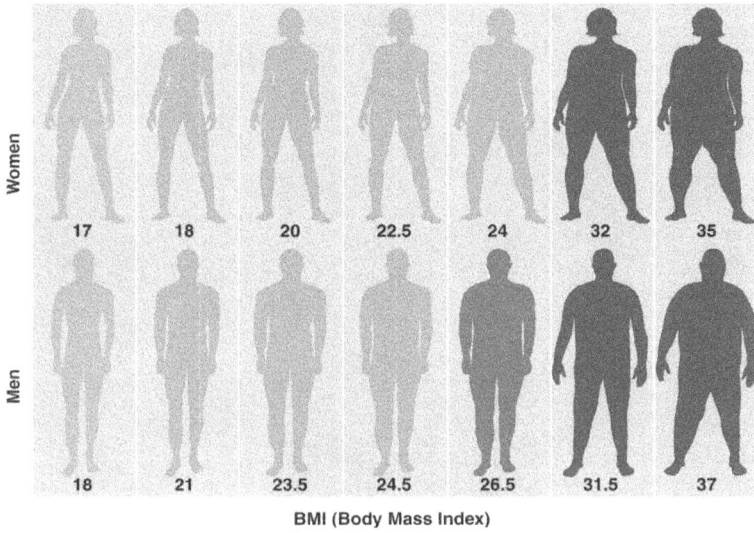

| Women | 17 | 18 | 20 | 22.5 | 24 | 32 | 35 |
| Men | 18 | 21 | 23.5 | 24.5 | 26.5 | 31.5 | 37 |

BMI (Body Mass Index)

GLUCUTCOACHING

B
THE JAPANESE LIFESTYLE

LIFE EXPECTANCY

The **Japanese Lifestyle** has the capacity to reverse obesity and pre-diabetes symptoms, and reduce glucose to normal levels by encouraging moderate eating and moderate activity. In doing so it enhances longevity.

According to a Japanese study, about 65% of participants in a trial were capable of reversing symptoms and glucose readings without the use of medicine.

In 2014, the life expectancy in Japan was **86 years for women and 80 years for men**. That is more than 6 more years of life for women and 5 more years for men than expected in America, and the longest worldwide.

Japanese people have the lowest obesity rate in the developed world: 3% of the total population. Compare that figure to 11% for the French and 32% for Americans (International Obesity Taskforce). The Japanese people are 10 times less obese than Americans on average—which is a good reason to adopt their diet. For those Japanese people who adopt characteristics of the western diet (fried food, carbohydrates, carbonated sodas, sweets, and juices, in large quantities), the average obesity rate rises to only 6%, which is attributed to the fact that even though they consume unhealthy foods, their quantities are still low compared to American consumption standards.

The average Japanese person eats 25%–50% fewer calories per day than the average American, which explains their lengthy lifespan. A Japanese person eats on average 1,000–1,500 calories instead of the 2000–2500 calories consumed by an average American.

My Japanese father-in-law runs 10 Km daily at the age of 76. Even with some deteriorating health conditions and a bad prognosis, he has overcome the odds, keeping his daily routine while skipping from his hospital bed to the amazement of his doctors.

FOOD and DIET
Japanese vs. Western Cuisine: Portions, Plate Size, Bento Box

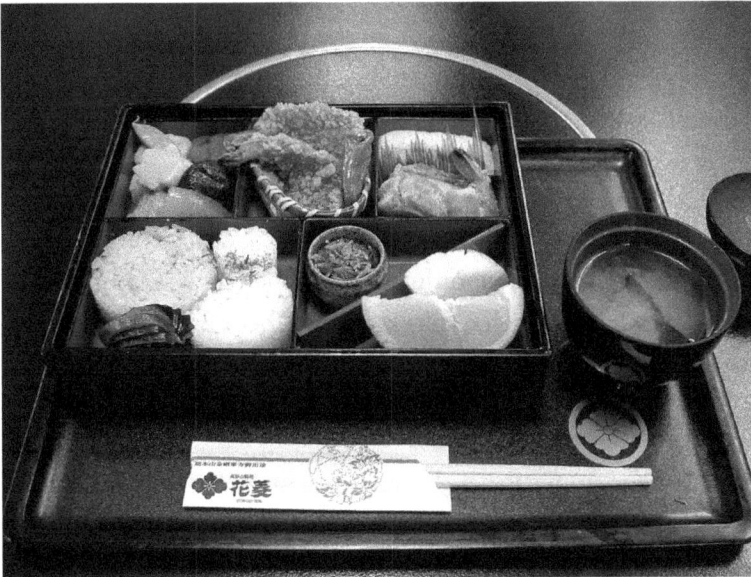

Bento Box—A combination of variety and low calorie

The Japanese diet is known worldwide. More Japanese restaurants are available than any other ethnic style. The Japanese consume about a third of the world's fishing production. The Japanese diet is low in fat, low in calories, fresh, natural, and high in protein content from fish, beans, and vegetables. This diet combines high quality products, and a home cooking culture that demands quality, natural products, High preparation standards, harmony and aesthetics in presentation.

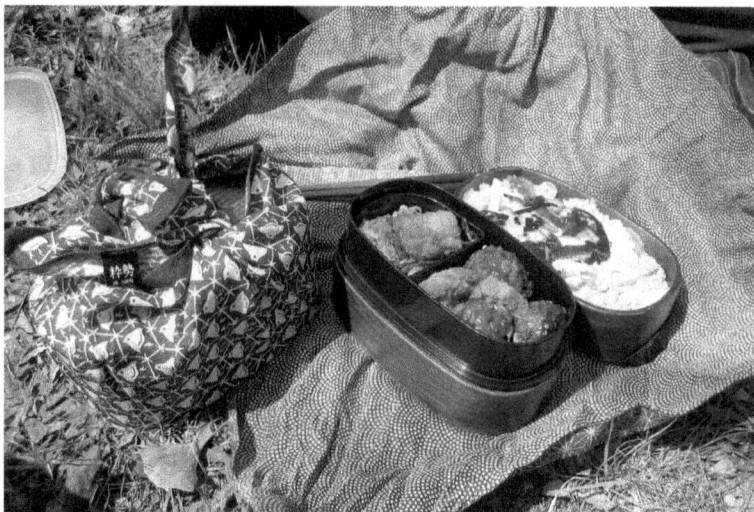

Japanese Picnic Meal—Bento Box Lunch – 400-500 calories

Japanese restaurants require chef certification, which comes after a period of 2 years training and subordination to a master. This structural society drives for perfection, which results in quality foods, excellent service, and a different eating experience based on aesthetic presentation and natural taste.

Presentation: Lacquered tray over wood base offers strong, settled colors.

Foods: All taken from Japanese harvest with in-season fruits and vegetables.

The Japanese Diet concentrates the energy from food into a compact and pleasurable size. The diet's healthy foundations are fish, vegetables and fruit; smaller portions; slow and mindful eating; with healthy additions like tofu and rice. From low to high-end eateries, presentation is an important aspect of dining. Small plates, decorations, and aesthetics are an integral part of the culture. These foundations are not found in western cuisine except in fancy restaurants that target the top 1% of the population.

Important Notice: The images shown offer examples of healthy Japanese cooking. These meals are based on an average of 500 Calories with low sodium and salt, low carbohydrates, low protein (100 grams), large quantities of fresh vegetables, healthy cooking (steamed, boiled), low sodium, low

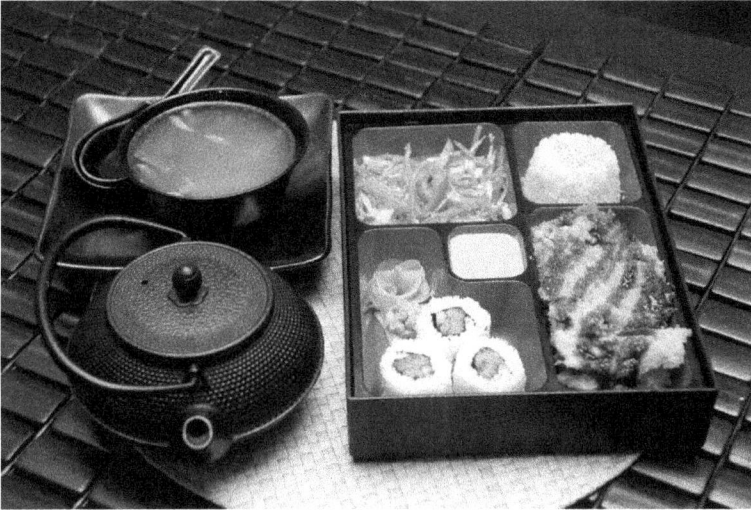

Sample for a 500-calorie meal

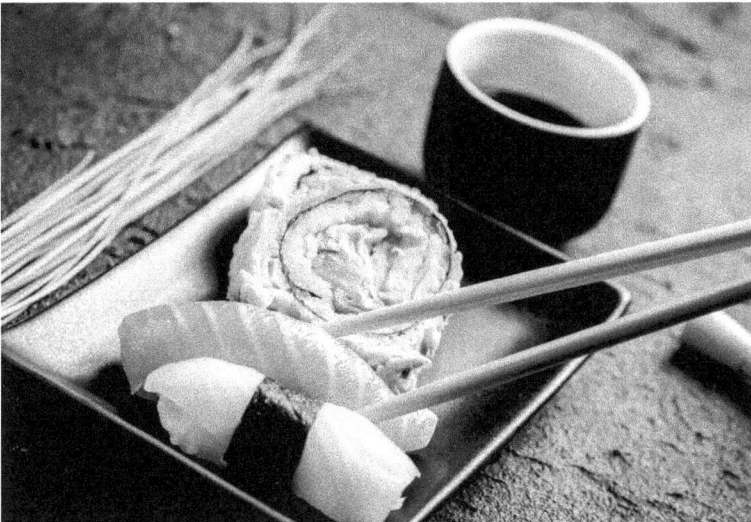

Low fat and low calories

quantities in general. Though the modern Japanese diet is high in sodium (soy and salt), the traditional Japanese diet contains such components only in minimal quantities. Japanese fast food contains foods fried in Canola oil, a very light oil which some dieticians associate with healthy cooking.

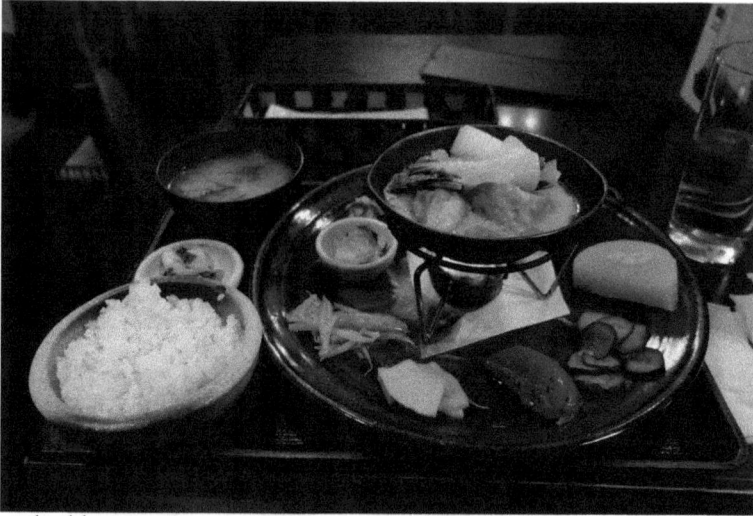

A healthy Japanese meal of about 500 calories I consumed in my favorite Osaka Restaurant

Caloric Intake—A secret to healthy eating is to replace energy-dense foods (containing a higher number of calories per gram) such as chocolate, potato chips, fries, and cookies, with those that are less energy-dense, like fruits, vegetables, and broth-based soups (a daily part of the Japanese diet).

In a study, women were served meals that were 25% smaller than average and contained 30% fewer calories according to the principles of energy density, eating an average of 800 calories less per day. They reported that they did not miss the extra food.

GLUCUTCOACHING Action Steps

Eat Non-filling Foods—Eat foods that fill, but don't add calories. For breakfast, consider oatmeal with fruits and nuts which provide large quantities of energy; this will fill you for half a day. Eggs will fill you as well.

Eat Smaller Portions—A survey conducted by The American Institute for Cancer Research (AICR) claimed that the quantity of food people were accustomed to eating was determined by the amount of food they placed on their plates.

It takes time to adjust your stomach to lower quantities. There is no quick fix to this issue, except for long periods of gentle acclimation. When I moved first to Japan in 2009, I complained repeatedly about the quantities I was served. Today, after over 5 years, I am accustomed to smaller plates. Having returned to the US, I often order only side dishes, and even then I cannot finish the served portions.

GLUCUTCOACHING Rule of Thumb

> Fill your stomach to 70-80%, which encourages the intestine to work properly, creates some slight feeling of residual hunger, and increases metabolism.

HEALTHY RECOMMENDATIONS

Over time these simple techniques will show significant results without you having to give up on the meal combination or attempt to change the chef's menu.

1. **Substitute white rice with brown rice**, a great whole-grain, and a high-fiber source of "healthy carbohydrates."

2. **Reduce sodium intake**, which is much higher in the Japanese diet because of the large amounts of soy sauce and pickled foods. Select lower-sodium miso, soy sauce, and teriyaki sauce. Chinese and Japanese populations have predominantly higher incidents of stomach cancer according to the Mayo clinic, and this is directly attributed to sodium (salt) intake.

3. **Replace large plates with smaller plates.** Store all the large plates and use only small ones when you prepare food

4. **Cut restaurant meals in half** and ask for doggie bags.

5. **Order side dishes only**. Usually, these are half the size of main courses. Ask the waiter for smaller portions, even when they don't appear on the menu.

6. **Request boiled/grilled foods** instead of fried foods.

Low Quantities and Quality over Size

The Japanese diet is known for small portion sizes and fresh, high quality ingredients. These are key points in pursuing a healthy lifestyle and balancing body weight.

GLUCUTCOACHING **Rule of Thumb**

> QQ – Control QUANTITY and QUALITY

Japanese Aesthetics

Japanese ceramics are an art form into themselves. The choice of ceramic utensils used in serving is given careful consideration; aesthetics are important. Over the centuries, this has contributed to a wide appreciation of the ceramic arts in Japan and worldwide. Japanese pottery is the result of continuous improvisation, experimentation, and refinement in the ceramic crafts. The older traditions of their pottery methods are still revered and practiced. Contemporary Japanese ceramicists are able to seamlessly merge modern elements of design, techniques, and materials with ancient traditions while maintaining the unique Japanese aesthetic embraced by modern trends in western culture.

The spread of Japanese cuisine has also contributed to increased numbers of people recognizing the cultural uniqueness of Japan and all the elements that contribute to it. The emphasis on high levels of food preparation and the aesthetics of food placement are all contributors to the fact that food **quantities** are less important than food **processes**.

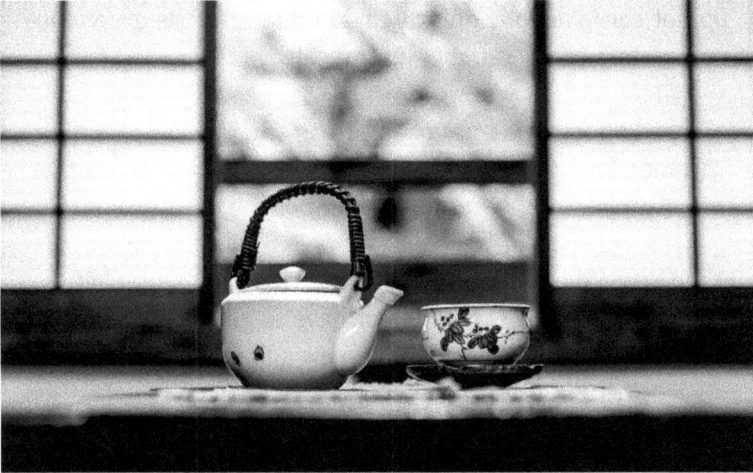

Ceramics—Small size and natural aesthetics present symbols from Nature (tree blossoms and bamboo leaves).

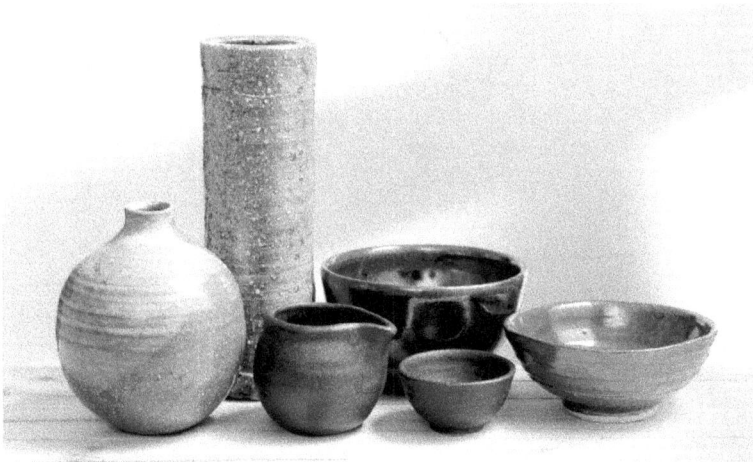

Quality Ceramics dishes are complementary accessories (offering a natural look). Choose aesthetics and beauty over quantity to make each meal a gratifying experience.

GLUCUTCOACHING **Rule of Thumb**

Do not consume food quickly and in quantity, the experience merely satisfies an unhealthy craving.

Consider food as a form of art, to be admired and savored. Arrange food on your plate by texture or color as a healthy offering to your body.

Find ways to elevate the eating experience into a reflective, aesthetic experience. You do not have to give up your love of food to be healthy. Instead, find new and more sophisticated ways to appreciate each meal.

CATEGORIES of JAPANESE ACTIVITIES
Minimal, Normal, Medium, Elevated, Athletic

Understand the differences between activity levels in order to track your activity accurately. **Metabolic syndrome is largely the result of being inactive**; one does not go from total inactivity to running 10 miles overnight.

By using the TANITA Monitoring instrument, you will be reminded of what you do during each day as the device records Activity Levels (METs) 24 hours a day, continuously 7 days.

Be aware of your current activity levels. Do not jump from Sedentary to Very Active but expand in moderation. This will prevent extensive stress, and will result in a higher probability that you'll continue the GLUCUT COACHING program.

Refer to the following levels of activity when using the monitoring system:

- **Minimal Survival Mode** – Sedentary; in bed; minimum amount of energy expended for heart function and to breath.

- **Normal Activity** – Minimal walking, driving, elevator riding, no exertion.

- **Medium Activity** – Walking 10,000 steps daily; walking up stairs instead of taking elevators; low intensity bicycle riding (for shopping); going to the gym 1–3 times a week; being conscious about activity.

- **Elevated Activity** – Running and walking 10 Km/day (about 4 miles); walking up stairs on all occasions; going to the gym every other day; bicycling 3 times a week; being conscious of activity and body movements at all times.

- **Athletic Activity** – All types of professional sports.

When my father-in-law stopped smoking at age 50, he started running daily in a runner's club with people 20–30 years younger. Now past his 75th year, he keeps this routine daily. He eats small meals based on the traditional Japanese diet. Retired, he travels periodically, climbs modest mountains, and enjoys a healthy life. His skin is as smooth as a 60-year-old man. His

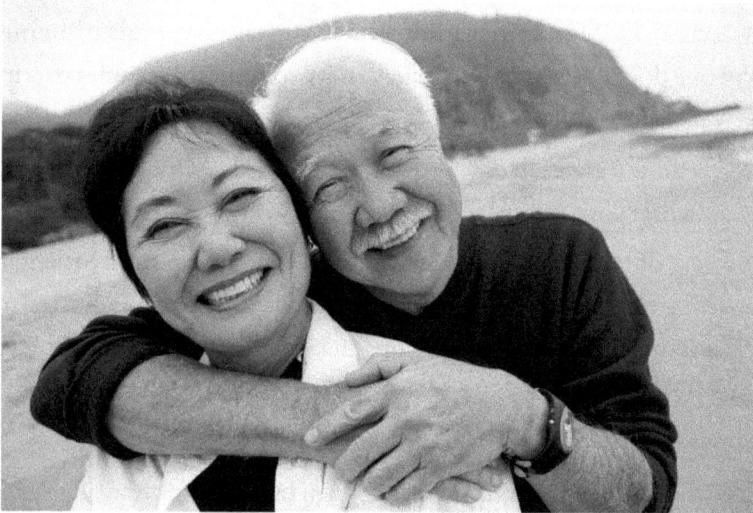

Retiree Jogging – a common practice

Metabolic Age shows 60-year-old readings. His energy level is high and he eats with a healthy appetite. It took him about 3 years to make this lifestyle a daily routine, which aligns with the theory that one needs 1–3 years to establish **Behavior Modification** that includes healthy eating based on the 500-calorie meal combined with exercise.

You Are Where You Live; You Are What You Eat

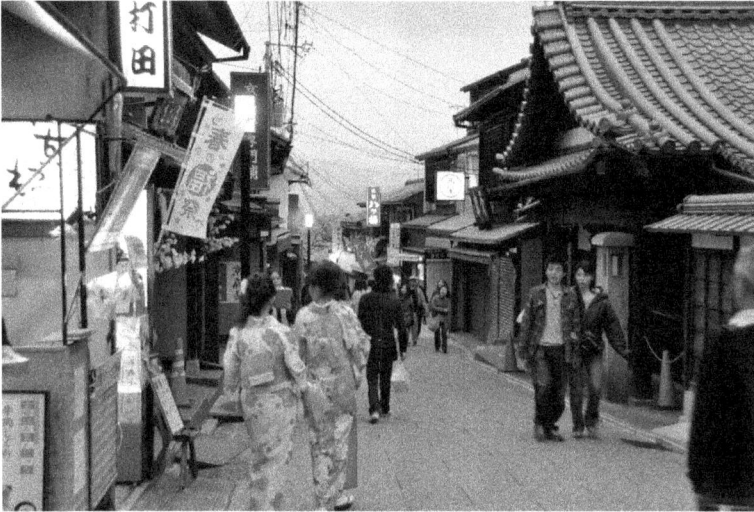

Urban Space — Street walks and community interactions

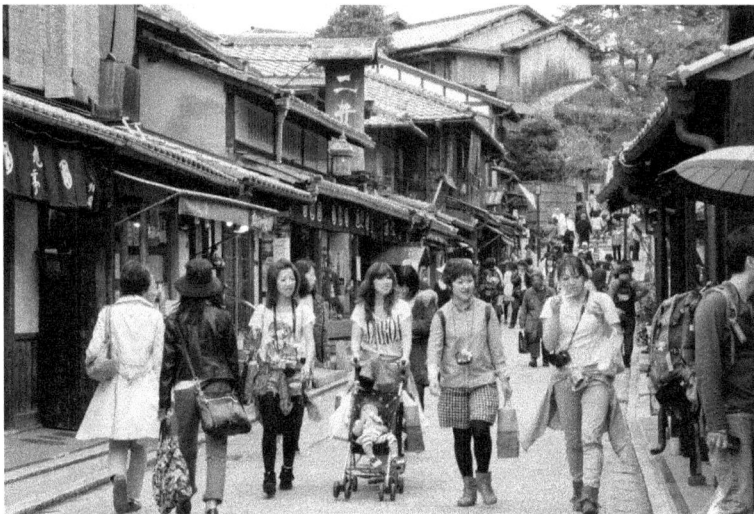

Shopping outdoors provides a personal experience and contributes to balanced social structures with modest body activity. Also, this type of outdoor shopping provides small vendors the benefits of being in business side by side with larger established companies that can afford to be in malls and shopping centers. As many of the vendors are old and close to retirement age, they might otherwise have difficulty finding employment, and become a burden on themselves and society.

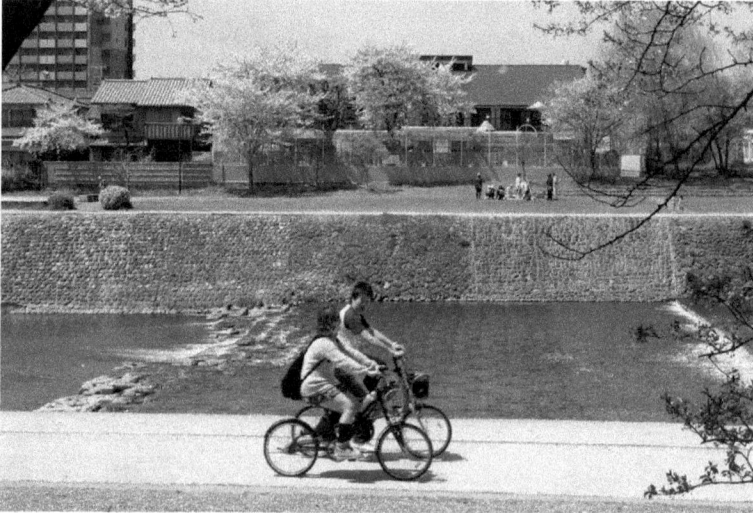

Japan offers an abundance of physical activities that are part of one's daily life. Those activities burn calories in a modest, natural way. Understanding how many calories you burn in your activities will help you determine how many calories you need to eat. Try using an online calorie calculator, such as http://www.caloriesperhour.com/index_burn.php to help you control calories. Enter the results into the GLUCUT COACHING tracking system (tables or app) and discuss the results with your healthcare provider.

IMPACT of LIFESTYLE on JAPANESE SOCIETY

Japan is an island nation with limited resources and a large population—all managing to live in harmony and peace. The country is Buddhist and has been influenced by Buddhist minimalism. Shizen, meaning "natural," is a core principle behind GLUCUT COACHING.

The Japanese tend to value small things over big things. This way of thinking evolved over thousands of years. It has both practical and religious roots.

Japan's preference for all things small shows up in dozens of ways:

- **Bicycling** – The Urban structure of Japan is such that it allows the extensive use of bicycles as a mode of transportation. Mothers cycle kids to school until age 6; elderly often bicycle until their 80s, increasing the health conditions of the general public.

- **Public Transportation** – Walking to and from the terminal may require hundreds or thousands of steps each day; taking stairs and avoiding elevators increases activity level.

- **Spring Mask** – facial filter masks are used extensively to avoid contracting viruses and exposure to smog

- **Small Thing Society** – Japan has a love for small things: small food portions (average 500 calories a meal), small houses (average 900 square feet for 3 bedrooms) with extensive energy cost reduction, minimal use of climate control, small hybrid cars, small gifts, etc.

- **Karaoke** – A form of relaxation after work that promotes social bonding
- **Onsen/Hot Springs** – A bath experience including body cleansing and ritual purification in a hot spring
- **Walking** – Shopping on the street level as opposed to in malls, walking to local parks/gardens
- **Tea Ceremony** – A place of relaxation and soul searching
- **Natural clothing** – High quality clothing made of natural materials
- **Macrobiotic food** – Food without contaminants / pesticides
- **Coffee Houses** – Places of relaxation and good social interaction / conversation
- **Massage chairs** – where one can get a relaxing massage at any time of day
- **Drinking Spring Water** – Extensive use of natural water resources. Our bodies contain 70% water. Because most of the contaminants found in public water systems cannot be removed, drinking spring water encourages longevity.

JAPANESE MACROBIOTIC FOOD

Macrobiotic food is another secret to staying healthy.

A macrobiotic diet emphasizes natural ingredients and is heavy on brown rice, beans, and fresh vegetables grown without artificial fertilizers. Foods to avoid are meats, dairy products, frozen and processed goods, and artificial sweeteners. The diet differs from vegetarianism in that it allows non-fatty types of fish and shellfish, as long as they are eaten occasionally. An interesting aspect of the macrobiotic trend in Japan is that it is taking place in the country where the macrobiotic diet originated.

The macrobiotic food theory developed in Japan between the end of the Edo Period in the 1860s and the early years of the Meiji Period that began in 1868 when some Japanese doctors started advocating the health benefits of their country's traditional cuisine.

Japanese Antioxidant Diet

Antioxidants are man-made or natural substances that may prevent or delay some types of cell damage caused by many foods, including fruits and vegetables and dietary supplements.

Examples of antioxidants include:

- Beta-carotene
- Lutein

- Lycopene
- Selenium
- Vitamin A
- Vitamin C
- Vitamin E

Vegetables and fruits (Japanese Diet) are rich sources of antioxidants. Eating a diet with lots of vegetables and fruits is healthy and lowers risks of certain diseases according to the National Institute of Health, National Center Complementary and Alternative Medicine.

Okinawa Diet

Residents of Okinawa, a southern Japanese island, are known for their **long life expectancy, high numbers of centenarians, and low risk of age-associated diseases**. Longevity is related to a healthy lifestyle, particularly to a traditional diet, which is low in calories yet nutritionally dense, with phytonutrients in the form of antioxidants and flavonoids. This diet calls for reduced intake of: meat, refined grains, saturated fat, sugar, salt, and full-fat dairy products.

ONSEN
The Japanese Hot Spring Experience

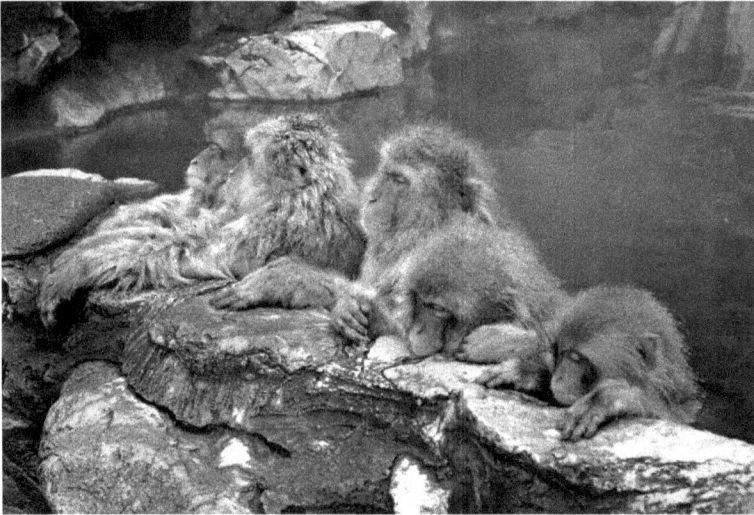

Onsen is an experience like no other: a bath, cuisine, and personal well-being experience—a holistic cleansing.

According to a Livestrong.com article, diet and exercise are the most effective ways to manage diabetes, but a new treatment of soaking in a hot bath is gaining recognition. "Diabetes Health" reported in a 2008 article, that Dr. Philip Hooper of the McKee 'l Center in Loveland, Colorado, conducted research for people with type 2 diabetes, and found that blood sugar levels decreased and sleep patterns were improved by daily hot tub therapy. Not all diabetes experts agree, and further study is needed, but with proper

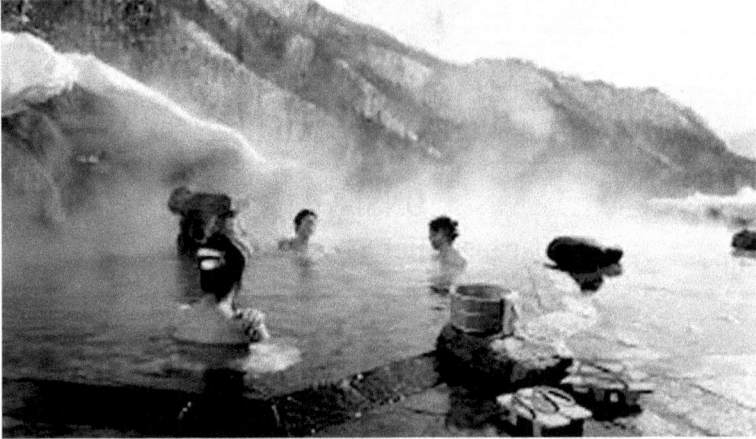

Social interaction – Communal living

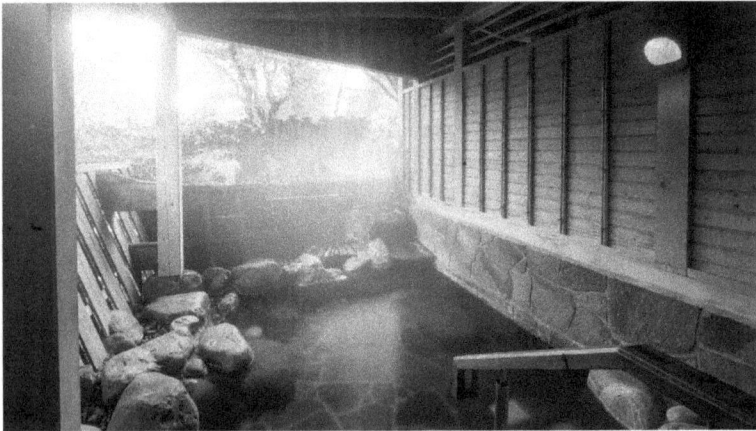

Seclusion and peace – an integral part of Japanese lifestyle where one is in touch with his own self

safety measures in place, diabetics can enjoy soaking in a tub and reap significant benefits.

An *onsen* is a Japanese hot spring and bathing facility that often includes the inns around the hot springs. As a volcanically active country, Japan has thousands of *onsens* scattered mostly throughout the countryside but also in cities. Traditionally used as public bathing places, onsens come in many types and shapes, including outdoor and indoor baths, publicly run by a

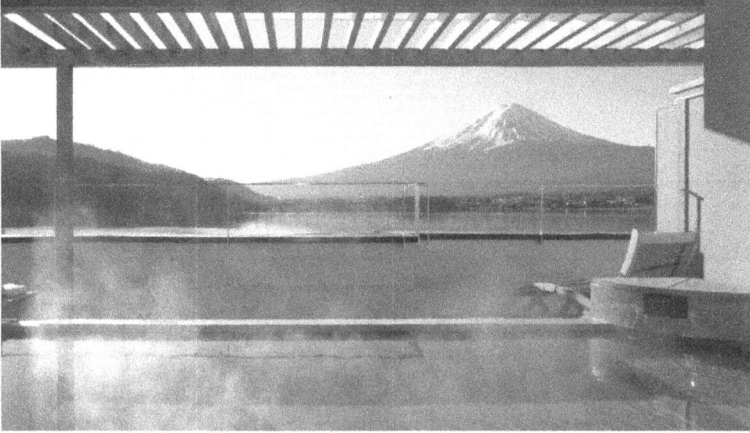

Nature and Health — Exposure to natural views and fresh air enhance the personal experience attributed to improved metabolism and wellbeing

municipality or privately run as part of a hotel, ryokan (traditional Japanese inn), or bed and breakfast.

Onsen are a tourist attraction that draws Japanese couples, families and company groups who want to get away from the hectic life of the city to relax. The Japanese often talk of the virtues of "naked communion" for breaking down barriers and getting to know people in a relaxed, homey atmosphere.

Onsen is not only a cleansing activity but a social interaction, reinforcing the inner self body, spirit, and soul.

Taking time to reflect is an essential part of the process of behavior modification. If you drive 100 miles per hour, you can't see the details along the road. You must walk, sweat, and feel hunger and pain before this lifestyle will became your second nature. The *onsen* experience—or some western substitute/equivalent—will help you in this process.

ONSEN HEALTH BENEFITS

Traditionally, *onsen* were located outdoors, but today they are mostly built indoors, using naturally hot water from geothermal heated springs. *Onsen* should be differentiated from *Sento*, indoor public bathhouses where the baths are filled with heated tap water. The legal definition of an onsen specifies that its water must contain at least one of 19 designated chemical elements, including radon and metabolic acid, and be 74°F (25°C) or warmer before being reheated. Stratifications exist for waters of different temperatures. Major onsen resort hotels typically feature a wide variety of themed spa baths and artificial waterfalls in the bathing area.

Onsen water is believed to have healing powers derived from its mineral content. A particular onsen may feature several different baths, each with water of a different mineral composition. The outdoor bathtubs are most often made from Japanese cypress, marble, or granite. Other services like massages may be offered.

The *Arima Onsen* is a rare hot spring that contains a lot of minerals and natural ingredients. It contains 7 different ingredients out of the 9 main ingredients designated to be included in medical treatment: simple hot spring water, carbon dioxide spring water, hydrogen carbonate, chloride, sulfate, ferruginous, sulfur, acid, and radioactive water springs (sulfur spring and acid spring are not included).

Health Benefits
- Soothes and relaxes muscles
- Relieves mental fatigue, releasing stress and tension

- Increases metabolic rate, providing a cardiovascular workout
- Improves blood circulation and relieves arthritic pain
- Cleanses skin and body of impurities; improves internal organ function
- Provides a relief from daily problems

Onsen—Hot springs are known to help alleviate the following conditions: sensitivity to cold, back problems, muscle and joint pain, skin problems,

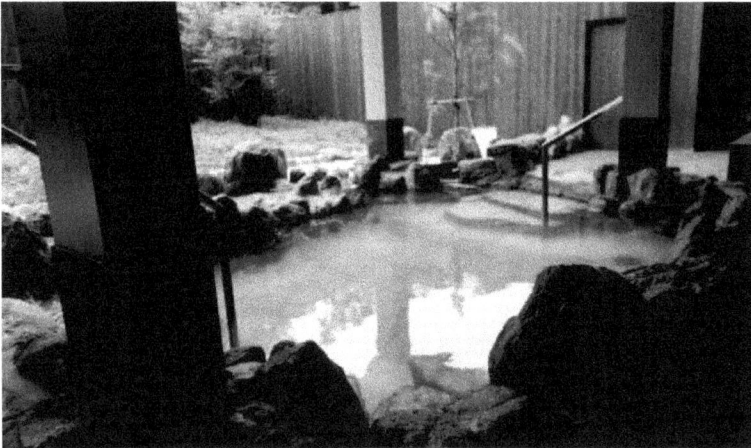

TOBA Onsen – *with pearl powder enhancement for skin perfection*

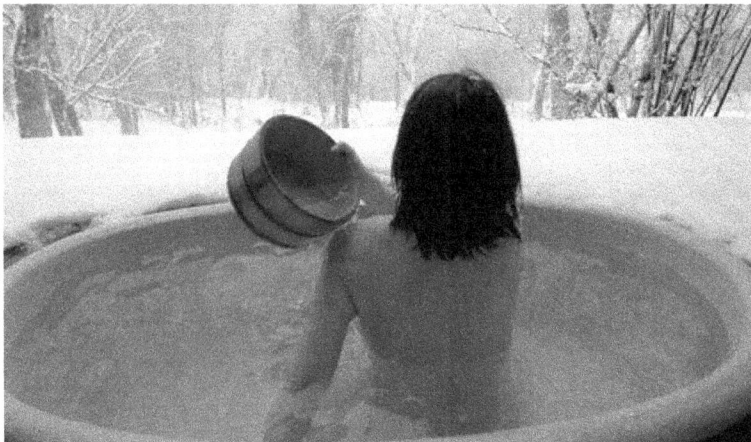

Nature and health merge into one

chronic eczema, antiseptic properties, allergic skin, hives, wounds, burn, rheumatism, high blood pressure, circulation in general but specifically arms and legs, degenerative joints, mild peripheral arterial disorder, menopausal discomfort, bronchial asthma, etc.

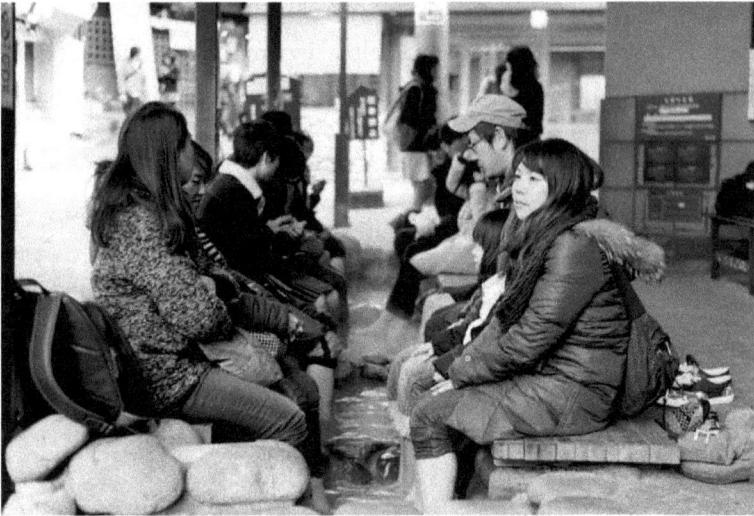

A high number of the onsen's *benefits are associated with the improvement of arterial disorders and blood circulation, both key contributors to diabetic disorders. The foot* onsen *shown above can enhance blood circulation.*

SOAKING UP THE HEALTH BENEFITS[1]:

Japanese scientists have been documenting the positive impact onsen can have on human health since the early eighteenth century.

Dr. Agishi's decades of studies have shown that hot spring water, depending on its mineral composition, can help people recover from certain surgeries and control a number of conditions, including rheumatism, neuralgia, hypertension and skin diseases.

---

1   Healing waters: The Japanese Onsen Experience - *Soaking up one of Japan's best-loved traditions is a tonic for both mind and body* - By C. James Dale 21 December, 2012

"There is a physiological mechanism of keeping the body temperature warm by some kinds of hot springs that differs from plain tap water," explains Agishi.

GLUCUTCOACHING Rule of Thumb

> Western alternatives: If you live in an area that offers natural hot springs, plan a visit. Otherwise, try a sauna or even a hot bath at home with bath salts and mineral you can add to the water.

Saunas—rooms with exceptionally high, dry heat and low humidity—top out at around 175-185F degrees. As you adjust to the temperature, your pulse rises by as much as 30 percent, increasing your blood circulation to aid muscle recuperation and improve flexibility. The persistent heat also fools your body into producing more white blood cells, boosting your immune system as it combats the perceived "fever." Excessive sweating purges your body of toxins[2].

Skin pores open up and allow the body to breath.

---

2   http://www.wapt.com/Can-post-workout-soaks-benefit-diabetics/15389714

C
THEORIES AND PRINCIPLES

URBANISM, ZONING, and HEALTH

What do urbanism, zoning laws have to do with your health? Obesity and Diabetes 2 are preventable if we reform the urban environment with good planning techniques combining public transportation, and walkable streets.

Though it is unlikely that you'll singlehandedly change the structure, layout, and priorities of your neighborhood town or city, it is valuable to understand that you are a product of your environment. Obesity, high blood sugar, and other health complications are a direct and natural result of a lifestyle that values convenience above all. Develop an awareness of how traditional western urban runs counter to the lifestyle your body was engineered for by thousands of years of natural selection. Find ways to compensate.

Modern America and the urban design framework that most affects our lives is based on the extensive use of the cars. We are accustomed to driving everywhere for the following reasons:

- **Distances** – Services are spread out and there's a lack of good public transportation.
- **Status** – The car becomes an extension of the owner, part of their identity, an expression of wealth.
- **Security** – It's more secure to exit your home garage and go underground to a parking garage than to wander the streets looking for a bus or cab.
- **Poor Public Transit** – It's more practical to rely on your own means

of transportation so you can control your schedule and place of connection (parking close to office compare to bus/train in a distance)

Urban Design

Living in Japan, an isolated Island with a secure environment and an abundance of good food (Japan imports very little food as freshness/quality is a key component of their diet), safety (no knifes or guns allowed in street), and reliable public transportation (extensive train and bus system), causes one to walk distances on a daily basis that would otherwise only be part of an exercise plan at the gym. An enlightened, planned cityscape environment forces consistent exercise because physical exertion is integral to the lifestyle.

Using the train/bus on a daily basis resulted in my walking more than 10,000 steps, the number recommended by healthcare professionals as the minimum daily activity level. Walking to and from my home to the train station, and taking the stairs rather than using the elevator greatly enhanced the amount of total exercise activity in my daily routine without requiring big changes or scheduling time at the gym.

Other healthy activities in this clustered urban environment include walking or riding a bicycle to shop or work, pick up the kids at school, go to the park, or visit the doctor.

Seek out opportunities to ride or walk as part of your routine. Look for safe, scenic routes through parks, woodlands, or quiet neighborhoods that add a touch of natural balance to your air-conditioned, regimented working life. Active Life can be enjoyable and easy while still burning calories, lowering blood sugar, and building muscle.

Carry foods bags from the market, and a bag with your computer and other accessory items such as books. Load your body with a "hidden" activity level that otherwise exists in a North American environment only when you visit the gym. By increasing the speed with which you walk to and from the train, run up and down the stairs, and so on, you can use the city as your own personal gym at zero cost and with zero wasted time.

The urban environment in Japan was created with pedestrian distances in mind, with residences located at an average of no more than a 500–1000-meter radius (1500 – 3000 feet) from a core center where the food market and commercial activities exist. This layout creates a clustered community with strong social ties, less reliance on motor transportation, and extensive use of bicycling and walking. The closer one is to the core, the smaller the streets become so they can only accommodate bicycles or very narrow cars (mini-cars).

With modern expansion and a high concentration of populations in contemporary cities, modern transportation harmonizes with the old urban cores by connecting the old centers with trains and subway systems, as humans cannot conveniently walk more than 2-3 km (about a mile or two) without the assistance of motor transportation. Even if you work far away and use the train, you still have the chance to move your body by walking each day to and from the train station, by shopping in the old core, and by using services (doctor, barber, school, etc.) within walking distance. Make moving and exercising your body part of your lifestyle. Sweat. Carry some weight. Breathe fresh air to engage the metabolic system.

Zoning

Zoning in Japan has resulted in a complete mixed-use environment. One can live in a house and be surrounded by small, ground floor shops selling anything from rice, cookies, and breads to services such as bicycle repair and medical care, and even low pollution factories, print shops, offices, etc. This urban design allows for a truly homogeneous city with a mix of accessible services tuned to supply and demand. Train stations lie in the heart of every neighborhood. These were historically built along the main roads connecting towns at the most concentrated cores with highest densities of pedestrian use. New development follows growth from those areas. An added benefit: trains are electric and don't pollute. A study in Japan shows that using the train saves 17 times as much energy as driving.

This type of zoning helps small business owners make ends meet after the mortgage has been paid off. Residents can remain in their homes during the golden years as services are nearby. This zoning helps maintain a close-knit society, where people know their neighbors and their customer's needs. In most cases, younger generations fix up or demolish old houses and build new ones on the same land their ancestors lived on.

The savings and value to society are not only realized through transportation savings associated with clustered activities, as one walks to buy bread or see the doctor, but also through a healthier, more secure, and supportive environment, where social stability is maintained over many generations. In the west we call it New Urbanism, but in fact it's an old way of living.

Another example I encounter in my life is modern Vancouver, which is considered by UN Habitat (2014 statistics) to be the 3rd most livable city in the world. Vancouver's new developments include new train stations; people prefer them to using their cars, saving resources and time. By contrast, this new urbanism is non-existent in Miami, and the results are evident: longer hours driving to work, clogged highways, and less quality of life overall. Neither to say, Miami is a wonderful city with fresh ocean air, great vistas seen from high bridges mostly or towers fronting the water, but the miss up is evident, If Miami was to be designed like NYC, then more urban access to water was evident, more recreational parks and boulevards with trees allowing room for bicycles paths would have made it a world class.

Urban Development: Problems and Solutions

2 examples that will highlight the problem and solution to density and urban Development:

Example 1

I am currently (2015) searching with investors for land in Miami's Little Havana neighborhood for the purpose of building affordable rental housing, where a vibrant Latin, blue-collar community lives. We are searching for land to build housing as the Brickell downtown corridor nearby is based on $3/SF rental rate, which is unaffordable to 80% of Miami population. A $1.2 -$1.5 $/SF affordability for this population segment can only be achieved with low cost housing built with a lower land cost, which is currently available at a 1 mile proximity to Brickell's new core at the Little Havana Neighborhood.

Most of Little Havana plots are 50'X150' Lots on average, and with the current Zoning Code of 1.5 Cars per unit, it makes the land not feasible to build on. Cars' requirements surpass the land space if to build to density, while the density achieved considering the parking makes the exercise of building unfavorable to Urban scape and walkable streets, with the Cars becoming the Main cause of the Problem / Solution.

Larger plots of land create the need for parking podiums and ramps, mostly exposed to street views. These diminish the street experience, deterring storefronts and lobby entries ,ultimately making streets unpleasant to walk, compared to an old urban scape, with pedestrian walkways and shops.

Walking = Healthy lifestyle = Vibrant community that was build with human scale in mind and not the automobile demands.

The Miami building code does not look behind the solution to the parking problem, creating with it a larger unnoticed social issue.

Example 2

I lived in Tel-Aviv in 1989, working with a Canadian development company that revolutionized the shopping experience in Israel by establishing indoor malls. That trend changed the old middle east open market experience to an indoor western experience with controlled environment that could only be accessed by car.

The problems with this type of mall are triple:

- The mall is a structural **box** inside the city that does not connect / interact with its surroundings
- **Controlled A/C** environment discourages sweating
- The **distances between establishments** is double as more merchandise requires larger stores, creating larger distances between the shoppers, with less eye contact and intimacy. This promotes quantities over quality. The old street market based on the Agora model developed in Greece that was part of the Old World environment for two millennia had only favorable components as it was based on proportions of the human scale. The New Urban Design movement is rediscovering this old scheme as a modern successful business model.

Neither to say, Diabetes is a major problem in Israel today.

CONCLUSION

A direct correlation exists between **Urban Design** and **Public Health**. The question is what the Government is willing to invest in **Public transportation** for quality of life or **Public Health** to battle the current results.

Cities are growing as societies are moving from agrarian culture to consumer culture. City cores are growing as well. Creating the right combinations of means of mobility, urban street spaces, and sustainable communities is the new bible for futuristic life.

The solution is found when we look at the issue as a whole. Solving only one component will be a waist of common resources and a cry for generations.

GLUCUTCOACHING Rule of Thumb

- **Vote with your feet.**
- **Live closer to work.**
- **Reduce your use of cars.**

- **Walk or use a bicycle**, saving valuable time while exercising at same time.

- **Carry a heavy handbag** daily and do more sweating and cardio exercise than weekly training in a gym in a steady way year around, while going to the gym require devoting time above your daily routine, with luck of consistency for the 80% of the population.

- **Live in a smaller but higher quality space** in order to lower living costs

- **Reduce Stress** by saving for non-rainy days (a major cause of Diabetes Type 2).

- **Live in proximity to neighbors**, the intimacy of the corner café, the breathing of natural air in the park as oppose to filtered air in an enclosed environment, and knowing your surroundings are all components that support us and give us comfort in our daily survival that cannot be acquired and replaced through any monetary means.

Japanese Health

Obesity, Pre-diabetes and Type 2 Diabetes are attributed first and foremost to lifestyle choices. The Japanese lifestyle has shown itself to be extremely healthy. This lifestyle combined with a low use of air conditioning and heating keeps metabolism at a more natural state, lowers energy costs, and contributes directly to the Sweat theory advocated by this book (see next section).

GLUCUTCOACHING Rule of Thumb

If possible, move to a city core where services are available in a contained area, such as a 3,000-foot radius. Avoid cars when possible and use a bicycle or walk instead.

JAPANESE HEALTH SYSTEM

My interaction with the Japanese Health system was minimal, but the sticking difference I noticed was the depth of detail I was encountered with.

As Japanese like small details and as explained at the beginning of this writing, by knowing the small details one can get to the heart of the problem, I encountered in my visits to the Diabetes doctors, several wall mounted boards that explain further the problem of Obesity and Diabetes.

図3　CTでわかる内臓脂肪面積

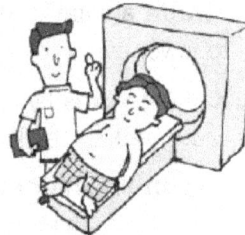

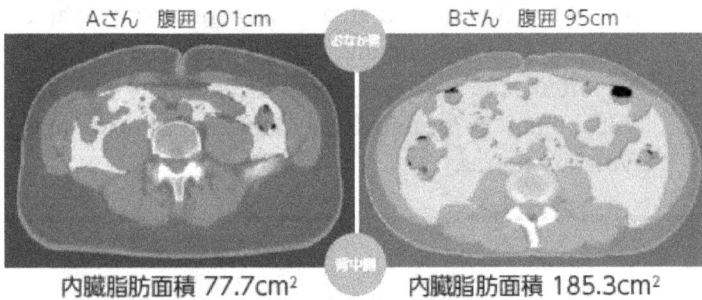

Aさん　腹囲 101cm　　　　Bさん　腹囲 95cm

内臓脂肪面積 77.7cm²　　　内臓脂肪面積 185.3cm²

同じ腹囲（86cm）なんですが・・・

皮下脂肪型肥満　　　　　　内臓脂肪型肥満

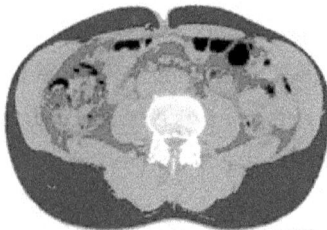

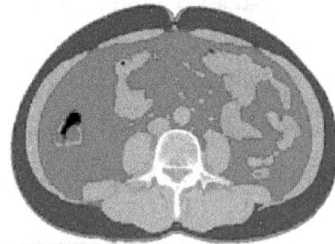

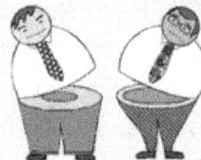

内臓脂肪　　50 cm²　　　　内臓脂肪　195 cm²
皮下脂肪 149 cm²　　　　　皮下脂肪 119 cm²

健康診断データ　　　　　　糖尿病・高尿酸血症
異常なし　　　　　　　　　治療中

Two similar circumference waist areas have two distinctly different visceral fat levels

The most valuable board visible was the Visceral fat. It shows clearly for two individuals with same waist circumference the internal Fat accumulated around the organs is key for a healthy condition.

A second board that made an impression was a Mammogram image of the vain showing clogging for those with high obesity levels.

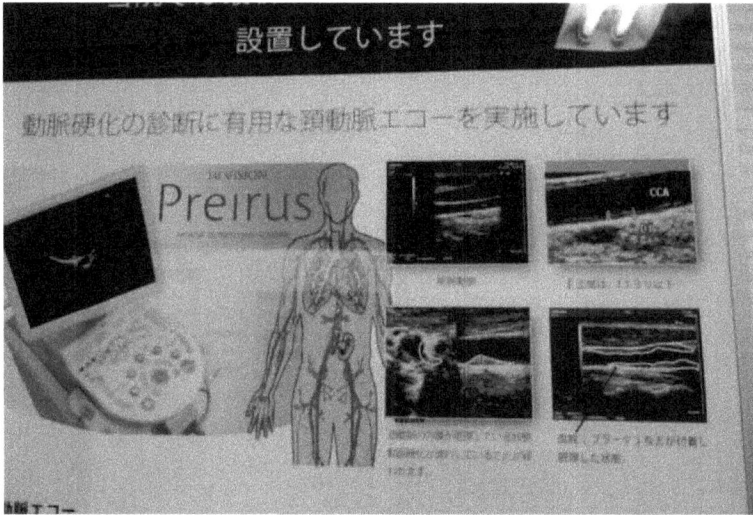

Traditional Japanese House: Old and Modern Form

Ando Tadao, a very famous Japanese Architect is most remembered by the "Row House in Sumiyoshi" (Azuma House, 住吉の長屋), a small two-story, cast-in-place concrete house completed in 1976, is an early work which began to show elements of his characteristic style. It consists of three equal rectangular volumes: two enclosed volumes of interior spaces separated by a third rectangular open courtyard. The courtyard's position between the two interior volumes becomes an integral part of the house's circulation system. The house is famous for the contrast between appearance and spatial organization which allow people to experience the richness of the space within the geometry, the natural light, air and outdoors when moving from one part to the other within the house, as one must cross an open bridge exposing oneself to the elements.

The size, space, courtyard, and propositions are all taken from the Old traditional Japanese house / row-house.

It's an extreme example, but that's why the natural living principle he advocates is most valuable. The traditional row house in Japanese culture has no air conditioning, natural air flow, steps to walk up and down, orientation to sun and light, and minimal dimensions.

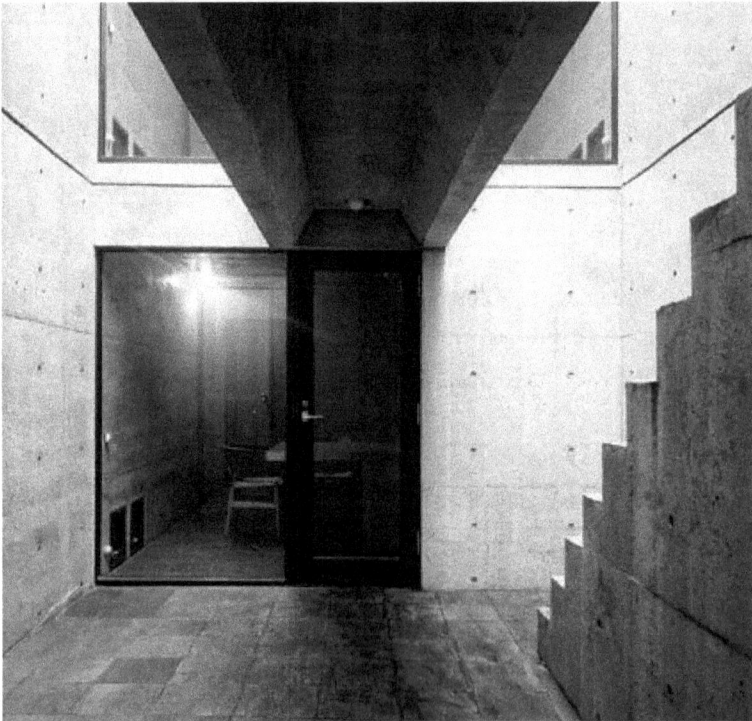

GLUCUTCOACHING **Rule of Thumb**

Think of your home as a place to retire and as a place to live. In your golden years, you will be most comfortable living in a space, neighborhood, and environment that promotes healthy, active living.

SWEAT THEORY

Sweating is good for you.

By allowing our bodies to sweat, we help the body to breathe through the skin, a natural function that has evolved over billions of years. As we have gained the ability to control much of our environment, we have been able to fix temperature levels through the use of air conditioning and heating at home, in the car, in the workplace, and even at entertainment venues. In doing so, we have impaired our metabolic systems, systems that do important work of cleansing toxins from the body and burning calories. The complete behavior of our body metabolism—how temperature changes relate to sweating—is not entirely understood by mainstream medicine. Further investigation is needed in order to evaluate the relationship between sweating and Diabetes.

Diabetes & Sweating Issues[1]

Diabetes may result in soaking night sweats.

Symptoms of diabetes include various issues concerning sweating and heat regulation.

Hypoglycemia and Sweating

Although diabetes is a disease caused by high levels of blood sugar, called hyperglycemia, patients with diabetes occasionally experience the opposite problem of low blood sugar, or hypoglycemia. Low blood sugar in diabetic patients is most often caused by medicines used to treat high blood sugar. Sometimes they work too well and cause blood sugar to drop to unhealthy levels. When people with diabetes experience a dip in blood sugar, the body releases epinephrine, also called adrenaline, in an attempt to raise blood sugar. In addition to the symptoms of shakiness and anxiety, epinephrine also causes the body to sweat profusely (National Diabetes Information Clearinghouse).

Looking at different bodily reactions—such as to extreme cold where the body reacts to hypothermia with an extreme rush of heat to protect and save itself—we can assume that this sweating caused without any exertion, in the case of Diabetes, is also an internal mechanism to energize the body, enhance blood circulation, clean toxins, and prevent blood clotting intended to restart a metabolic system that is shutting down.

The consequences of inactive modern living that leads to not sweating for long periods is a subject that needs further investigation.

Why It's Important to Sweat

The main reason our bodies sweat is to cool down. Evaporation of water on the skin cools the body. However, perspiration also plays an important role in the excretion of toxins and waste products.

Variations in the Chemical Composition of Sweat

The chemical composition of sweat varies from individual to individual. It also depends on what they have been eating and drinking, why they are sweating, how long they have been sweating, and on several other factors.

Perspiration consists of water, minerals, lactate, and urea. On average, the mineral composition is:

- sodium (0.9 gram/liter)
- potassium (0.2 g/l)
- calcium (0.015 g/l)
- magnesium (0.0013 g/l)

Trace metals the body excretes in sweat:

- zinc (0.4 milligrams/liter)
- copper (0.3–0.8 mg/l)
- iron (1 mg/l)
- chromium (0.1 mg/l)
- nickel (0.05 mg/l)
- lead (0.05 mg/l)

Air Conditioning and The Psychometric Chart

The Psychometric Chart below illustrates a scientific perspective on indoor and outdoor air conditions, and how they relate to human thermal comfort. It details general room temperature and humidity requirements needed for the body to stop sweating and to feel comfortable. This chart was designed when air conditioning was first introduced. Air conditioning has existed since the time of the ancient Egyptians in the form of Desert ventilation when warm air was directed through large chimneys over cold water reservoirs with the air temperature cooled down called Evaporative Coolers, but only in the 1950s did Electric A/C become common in households with the invention of the heat pump and coolant refrigerants.

There are many ways to heat or cool an environment, the most important element is having in mind a designer that consider Green solutions.

When you start sweating naturally on a regular basis, you will see a **reduction in blood sugar levels, better blood circulation, more stami-**

na/body energy, and loss of weight. Slowly increase sweating levels by increasing your level of activity. Always check with your healthcare provider before making changes.

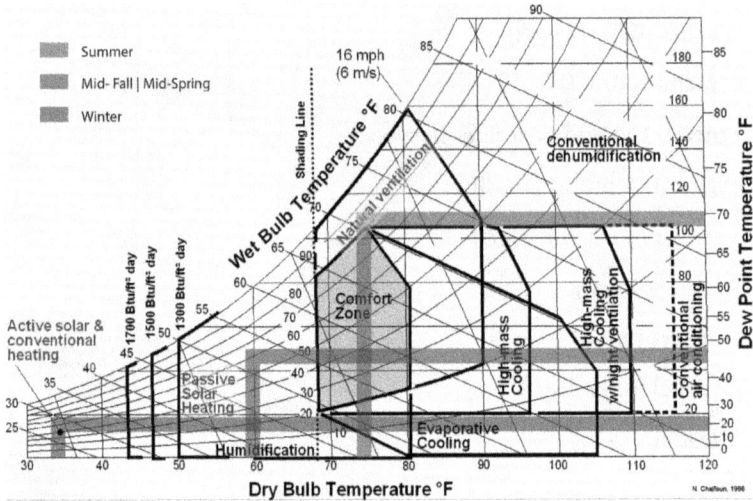

Avoid air-conditioning and heating systems as much as possible. Cooling of the human body through perspiration as shown on the Psychometric Chart (wet-bulb temperature and absolute humidity) as the heat of the surrounding air increases in summer is essential to a healthy life. Other mechanisms may be at work in extreme winter or summer using such mechanism as humidity or "damp cold."

On Sweating and Not Sweating

THE GOOD

Sweating burns fat throughout the body, in all areas. Sweat is good for the skin. Water hydrates, minerals and salt naturally exfoliate, and urea and uric acid combat dry skin and dermatitis. Sweating purges the skin of bacteria, dirt, oils, and impurities. The optimal pH factor for the skin is the same as the pH factor of sweat.

Sweating is a signal during exercise that the warm-up phase is over, and you are entering your performance zone. When you are in your performance zone, sweat regulates your body temperature and signals your body's ability to hydrate. Walking 10,000 steps in a day is not the same as walking the same distance in one hour. The difference will show in your indicators when you fill out the GLUCUT COACHING tables.

THE BAD

Impurities flushed out when you sweat can stay on your skin. When your skin begins to re-absorb them, pH factors change and this can lead to irritation and rash. The sweat expelled through the apocrine glands in the skin is responsible for that familiar post-workout body odor.

What's not entirely clear is the impact of not sweating on internal organs. Few if any studies have addressed the impact, and no papers have been written on the effects. We know about fatty livers as result of fatty foods. We also know about fat around the heart, but we really don't know what the effect is when the metabolism is inhibited as result of not sweating and low activity.

GLUCUT COACHING asserts that sweating is essential for good metabolism. It helps reduce blood sugar levels, increases heart strength, cleanses toxins, causes better bowel discharge, creates positive emotional states, increases longevity, enhances sex drive, helps maintain body weight, and strengthens the body against diseases. Extensive documentation supports this claim. As we are not Health care providers, we can only emphasize on the subject and not make direct recommendations. Seek advice from your healthcare provider.

The Japanese Sweating/Cleansing technique

Japanese people go to onsens and take baths daily. The baths are heated to 105°F(41°C) and are taken for 10 minutes or so, raising their heart rates, increasing sweating, and cleaning their pores. They repeat the process 3–4 times. Afterward, bathers feel their metabolic rates increase. Their skin is clean and their pores are open. These results are similar to those produced by the sweating process.

> **Sweating is an essential GLUCUT COACHING technique**

Supporting for Sweating Theory

DIABETES & SWEATING ISSUES, MATTHEW BUSSE, LIVESTRONG.COM

Low blood glucose due to diabetes may result in soaking night sweats. Symptoms of diabetes include various issues concerning sweating and heat regulation.

HYPOGLYCEMIA AND SWEATING

When people with diabetes experience a dip in blood sugar, the body releases epinephrine, also called adrenaline, in an attempt to raise blood sugar. In addition to the symptoms of shakiness and anxiety, epinephrine also causes the body to start sweating profusely.

INABILITY TO SWEAT

One frequent effect of diabetes is damage to the nerves connecting the brain to the rest of the body, which is called diabetic neuropathy. If the nerves that control sweat glands are damaged, they may not be able to activate the sweat glands and produce sweat. This inability to sweat is called anhidrosis. One study published in Mayo Clinic Proceedings found that 94 percent of patients with diabetic neuropathy had abnormalities in their abilities to sweat. People who cannot sweat often have trouble regulating their body temperature because sweat helps the body to cool down. As a result, diabetic patients with anhidrosis may easily become overheated in warm temperatures or after physical exertion.

Excess Sweating

Some patients with diabetic neuropathy experience the opposite effect. When the nerves that control the sweat glands are damaged; they sweat too much (University of Washington Department of Medicine). Diabetic neuropathy has been linked to excess sweating, particularly at night or while eating. Some patients may wake up in the middle of the night because their sheets are drenched in sweat, which is sometimes referred to as "soaking night sweats."

Living for long periods in a temperature-controlled, air-conditioned environments prevents us from sweating normally and directly impacts the nervous system. The nervous system is critical for our bodies to function normally and regulate the sweat. The impacts of constant temperatures on the nervous system indirectly affect our blood circulation and our sugar processing, which can result in a pre-diabetes and later on type 2 diabetes metabolic malfunction.

Sweating is important, not just for normal blood circulation, but for balancing the nervous system and the health of the hypothalamus based in the center of our brain (see below).

Looking back at the Dry Bulb temperature graph, moving away from the comfort zone of 20-21C degree (+/-71 Fahrenheit) for longer periods may reverse symptoms of pre-diabetes and type 2 diabetes, including abnormal blood sugar readings, nervous system impairment, weight increase, etc.

Disclaimer: This theory has not been proven in a lab or through a medical trial. It is based only on my observations, research, and personal experience.

Hypothalmus – The Gland in the Brain that Controls Sweat

Sweating allows the body to regulate its temperature. Sweating is controlled by the hypothalamus where thermo-sensitive neurons are located. The heat-regulatory function of the hypothalamus is affected by temperature receptors in the skin. High skin temperature reduces the set point for sweating and increases the gain of the hypothalamic feedback system in response to variations in core temperature. The sweating response to a rise in 'core' temperature is much larger than the response to the same increase in average skin temperature.

What this tells us is that by shutting down the body's internal sweat cycle, we shut down the metabolic mechanism of organs in the body. This probably affects other metabolic functions such as blood sugar cycles. We

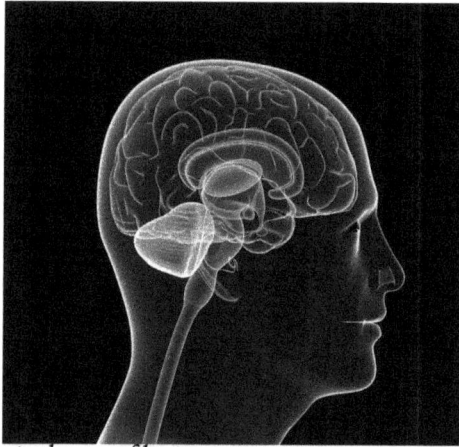

Hypothalamus in the core of brain

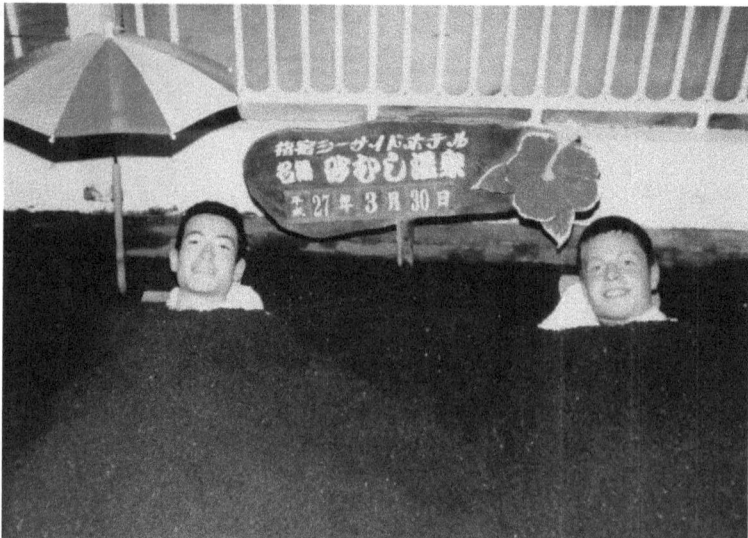

Sand Onsen — Another Japanese innovative way to elevate body heat and sweat

know that in the morning, glucose readings (fasting blood sugar level) are typically lower than in the later hours (called "dawn effect"). We may well be shutting down our ability to burn fat, which works against our self-cleansing cycle.

GLUCUT COACHING focuses on targeting the metabolic system with Healthy Food, Activity (Sweat), and Motivation.

GLUCUTCOACHING

D
MONITORING SYSTEM

MONITORING YOUR LIFESTYLE

Monitoring blood sugar is western medicine's main tool for keeping pre-diabetes under control. By testing your blood sugar, you can determine your blood glucose level at any time. Ask your healthcare provider how many times a day you should check your blood sugar levels. Many people check their blood sugar levels multiple times each day, at fasting in the morning (after sleep and before breakfast), before and after eating (2 hours after). Remember the cost: over $1 per test.

But measuring blood sugar alone is not going to alleviate your problem. Your healthcare provider will scrutinize your blood sugar readings in depth, but it is less likely that your diet or exercise patterns will get the same scrutiny. GLUCUT COACHING recommends holistic monitoring. **Only by monitoring all of the elements of your lifestyle** can you say positively that you are doing everything you can to fight your condition. This means following a monitoring protocol.

Self-monitor on a daily, weekly, monthly, and yearly basis. Without monitoring, you lose perspective on your changes. You can track your progress in many ways: taking pictures, writing in a notebook, making entries in computer spreadsheet, relying on the assistance of family and friends, or by using the GLUCUT app.

The GLUCUT COACHING program will assist you with recording, advising, and following up with recommendations throughout the program as you progress in making lasting behavioral changes.

Short Term Monitoring

Monitor blood sugar, activity levels, and calories daily.

- **Blood Sugar** – Check blood glucose every day, before and after every meal in the initial stages to evaluate how different foods affect your blood sugar levels. Once familiar with each food and its impact, you can move to monitoring once a day at fast. Share the results with your healthcare provider.

- **Activity Level** – Stay active every day to stay conscious about the benefits of exercise and body activity. Talk with your healthcare provider about increasing your level of activity.

- **Calories** – Take control of what you eat by tracking your calories every day. Allow for some breaks and moments of encouragement. Your BMR (Basal Metabolic Rate – the minimum number of calories you need to survive without activity) is taken when you start the program and it upgrades as your weight changes. The TEE (Total Energy Expenditure – the number of calories you burn in a day) is calculated depending on your activity levels; you can calculate it yourself with the formulas provided in this book or use one of the recommended monitoring devices.

When you monitor your diet and exercise, the results of your lifestyle changes and overall health will be evident.

GLUCUT COACHING is about increasing your daily activity level without making drastic changes in your daily life and schedule. This idea makes it more likely for you to make lasting changes in your daily life. This is one reason we call our method a lifestyle behavior modification approach.

Long Term Monitoring

Use the following 5 (FIVE) monitoring categories to track your progress: Personal Data, Key Health Indicators, Body Composite, Activity, and Weekly Summary.

PERSONAL DATA

Item	How to Measure	Interval
Age	Self-measurement	When starting program
Height	Self-measurement	When starting program
Weight	Tanita/prof. Fitscale Weight	Periodically
Body Fat %	Tanita/ prof. Fat Fitscale	Weekly
Stride Length	Self-measured; 10 steps divided by length	When starting program
Physique	Tanita Weight – Fitscale weight	Periodically
BMR	Tanita Hand Monitoring – Fitscale Weight	Periodically
BMI	Table or Search Web /Computer	Periodically
Visceral Fat	Mid-body fat /waist, Tanita Fitscale	Periodically

KEY HEALTH INDICATORS (HEALTHCARE PROVIDER ASSISTANCE)

Item	How to Measure	Interval
A1C	Blood test (usually performed by healthcare provider)	3 Months
Glucose	Monitor at Fast	Daily
LDL	"Bad" cholesterol (Blood Test)	3 Months
HDL	"Good" cholesterol (Blood Test)	3 Months
Blood Pressure	Blood circulation	Weekly
Heart Rate	Heart Health	Daily
Sleep Monitoring	Self-analyze sleep Activity	Daily
Body Temperature	Analyze Healthy body	Weekly / Monthly

Body Composite (TANITA FITSCALE or Similar)

Item	How to Measure	Interval
Weight	Will adjust BMI readings (Scale at Fast)	Daily
Height	Measure your height with initiation	With program initiation
BMR – Basal Metabolic Rate	Calories needed daily to survive (minimum intake)	Daily (Scale) or calculate once
Metabolic Age	Compare your physical stage to others (Scale)	Weekly
Body Fat	Will Monitor Body Fat (Scale)	Daily
BMI	Body Mass Index – Weight to Height (Table / Auto calc.)	Daily
TEE (Alternate measure)	Weigh Weight X 12 (another way of Intake) (BMR X Factor) (Self calculated) TANITA AM120E	Daily
AEE – Activity Calories Consumed	Total Calories burned through the Day	Daily
Waist	Measure your fat at waist	Weekly
Visceral level	Fat at body Waist level (Tanita)	Daily / Weekly

Activity

Item	How to Measure	Interval
Energy Levels	1-Low, 2-Medium, 3-High	1 Week (Self)
Activity Levels Factor	Sedentary: 1.2 Low-Active: 1.35 Active: 1.55 Very Active: 1.7 Extreme : 1.9 BMR X Factor = Calories Needed for balance energy levels	Daily (Self) BMR X Factor = Calories Needed for balance energy levels
Pedometer	Distance of Walking/Running/Steps (Tanita monitor)	Daily—Self

Sex Activity	Energy levels (Self-measurement)	Weekly
Activity/Walk/ Run	3Km walk, 5Km walk, 1 Km run(TANITA)	Daily
Speed/Walk/Run	4 Km/h , 6 Km/h, 10 Km/h(TANITA)	Km/Hour
Calories Burned	Tables / Internet (Calc.)	During Exercise
Sweat	Dry / Light /Mid Wet/ Wet / Pouring (Self measurement)	Daily

WEEKLY SUMMARY (EXAMPLE)

Item	Results	Notes
Weight	165 Lb	Lower 13Lb
BMI	27.5	Lower 2 point
Body Fat	22.5%	Overweight by 10%
Glucose Average	160	Lower to 120
Calories Needed	1950 (Daily)	BMR X Factor or TEE
Calorie Intake	2200 (Average Daily)	Eat less / Change diet
Activity Level	Moderate	Raise Activity Level
TEE	1850	Lower 200 Calories a day
Sweat Level	4 Levels correspond to Activity Levels	Increase Activity Levels

HEATH CORRELATIONS

Monitoring reveals interesting correlations between health measurements:

- Number of **calories consumed** versus **calories needed** to maintain healthy body
- Body fat versus carbohydrates
- Activity level versus visceral reading Levels
- Blood sugar levels versus sweat levels
- General energy versus overall health

Calorie Count – Relates to energy levels and fat reduction. Your readings will eventually show improvement in BMI, Body fat percentage, and Energy levels.

Pedometer Activity (Walking only) – Relates to blood sugar levels and sweating conditions. Your glucose readings will be lower immediately after activity, and in the long term will lower your AIC.

Sweat Levels – Relate to predictive values for sedentary, light, moderate, and vigorous categories. The more you sweat, the better the glucose levels you will read.

Body Mass Index (BMI)

As explained before, the BMI is an indication of your obesity level. Your BMI score allows you to compare your own visceral (waist) area to other individuals of different heights and weights. Monitor your BMI at all times; watching your BMI drop will motivate you to continue following the GLUCUT COACHING program.

BMI is calculated the same way for both adults and children. However, the average BMI - body mass indices for men and women are quite different.

Description	Women	Men
Essential fat – Minimum	10–13%	2–5%
Athletes	14–20%	6–13%
Fitness	21–24%	14–17%
Average	25–31%	18–24%
Obese	32%+	25%+

CALCULATING YOUR BMI

Measurement Units	Formula and Calculation
Pounds and inches	Formula: weight (lbs.) / [height (inches)]2 x 703 Calculate BMI by dividing weight in pounds (lbs.) by height in inches (in) squared and multiplying by a conversion factor of 703. Example: Weight = 150 lbs., Height = 5'5" (65") Calculation of BMI: [150 ÷ (65)2] x 703 = 24.96

You can also use an online BMI Calculator, such as the one at the National Heart, Lung, and Blood Institute: http://www.nhlbi.nih.gov/health/educational/lose_wt/BMI/bmi-m.htm

INTERPRETING BMI FOR ADULTS

For adults 20 years and older, BMI is interpreted using standard weight status categories that are the same for all ages and for both men and women. For children and teens, the calculation of BMI is age and sex specific.

Standard weight categories associated with BMI ranges:

BMI	Weight Status
Below 18.5	Underweight
18.5 – 24.9	Normal
25.0 – 29.9	Overweight
30.0 and Above	Obese

The following chart shows weight ranges, corresponding BMI ranges, and weight status categories for a sample height of 5'-9".

Height	Weight Range	BMI	Weight Status
	124 lbs. or less	Below 18.5	Underweight
	125 lbs. to 168 lbs.	18.5 to 24.9	Normal
5' 9" (sample)	169 lbs. to 202 lbs.	25.0 to 29.9	Overweight
	203 lbs. or more	30 or higher	Obese

It takes the average person 1–3 years to adjust behavior and stomach size, and lose weight to attain normal/healthy BMI levels. Be patient with yourself.

WEIGHT lbs	100	105	110	115	120	125	130	135	140	145	150	155	160	165	170	175	180	185	190	195	200	205	210	215
kgs	45.5	47.7	50.0	52.3	54.5	56.8	59.1	61.4	63.6	65.9	68.2	70.5	72.7	75.0	77.3	79.5	81.8	84.1	86.4	88.6	90.9	93.2	95.5	97.7
HEIGHT in/cm	Underweight					Healthy						Overweight					Obese					Extremely obese		
5'0" - 152.4	19	20	21	22	23	24	25	26	27	28	29	30	31	32	33	34	35	36	37	38	39	40	41	42
5'1" - 154.9	18	19	20	21	22	23	24	25	26	27	28	29	30	31	32	33	34	35	36	36	37	38	39	40
5'2" - 157.4	18	19	20	21	22	22	23	24	25	26	27	28	29	30	31	32	33	33	34	35	36	37	38	39
5'3" - 160.0	17	18	19	20	21	22	23	24	24	25	26	27	28	29	30	31	32	32	33	34	35	36	37	38
5'4" - 162.5	17	18	18	19	20	21	22	23	24	24	25	26	27	28	29	30	31	31	32	33	34	35	36	37
5'5" - 165.1	16	17	18	19	20	20	21	22	23	24	25	25	26	27	28	29	30	30	31	32	33	34	35	35
5'6" - 167.6	16	17	17	18	19	20	21	21	22	23	24	25	25	26	27	28	29	29	30	31	32	33	34	34
5'7" - 170.1	15	16	17	18	18	19	20	21	22	22	23	24	25	25	26	27	28	29	29	30	31	32	33	33
5'8" - 172.7	15	16	16	17	18	19	19	20	21	22	22	23	24	25	25	26	27	28	28	29	30	31	32	32
5'9" - 175.2	14	15	16	17	17	18	19	20	20	21	22	22	23	24	25	25	26	27	28	28	29	30	31	31
5'10" - 177.8	14	15	15	16	17	18	18	19	20	20	21	22	23	23	24	25	25	26	27	28	28	29	30	30
5'11" - 180.3	14	14	15	16	16	17	18	18	19	20	21	21	22	23	23	24	25	25	26	27	28	28	29	30
6'0" - 182.8	13	14	14	15	16	17	17	18	19	19	20	21	21	22	23	23	24	25	25	26	27	27	28	29
6'1" - 185.4	13	13	14	15	15	16	17	17	18	19	19	20	21	21	22	23	23	24	25	25	26	27	27	28
6'2" - 187.9	12	13	14	14	15	16	16	17	18	18	19	19	20	21	21	22	23	23	24	25	25	26	27	27
6'3" - 190.5	12	13	13	14	15	15	16	16	17	18	18	19	20	20	21	21	22	23	23	24	25	25	26	26
6'4" - 193.0	12	12	13	14	14	15	15	16	17	17	18	18	19	20	20	21	22	22	23	23	24	25	25	26

Quick Reference BMI Chart

Body Fat

Body fat percentage is the total mass of fat divided by total body mass. Body fat can be categorized as either essential body fat or storage body fat.

Essential body fat is necessary for maintaining life and reproductive functions. The percentage of essential fat is 3–5% in men, and 8–12% in women.

The percentage of essential body fat for women is greater than that for men, due to the demands of childbearing and other hormonal functions.

Stored body fat protects our internal organs. The minimum recommended total body fat percentage is higher than that of the essential fat percentage. You can determine body fat percentage by measuring with calipers or by using bioelectrical impedance analysis—your TANITA Weight.

Body fat percentage is a measure of your fitness level. It is the only body measurement that directly calculates a person's relative body composition without regard to height or weight. The widely used Body Mass Index (BMI) allows the comparison of the visceral (waist) area of individuals with different heights and weights. While BMI largely increases as visceral fat increases due to differences in body composition, other indicators of body

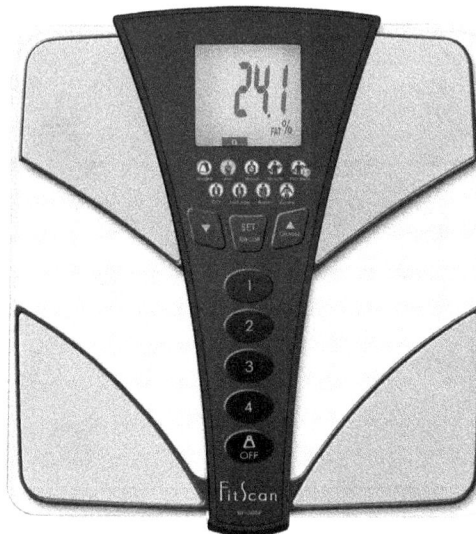

TANITA BC-585 Fit Scale

fat give more accurate results. For example, individuals with greater muscle mass or larger bones will have higher BMI.

The TANITA Scale will measure: **weight, body fat, metabolic age, visceral fat, body water %, muscle mass, physique rating, DCI/ BMR, metabolic age, and bone mass**.

Equivalent machines exist in the marketplace and should be evaluated for their number of indicators and specifications.

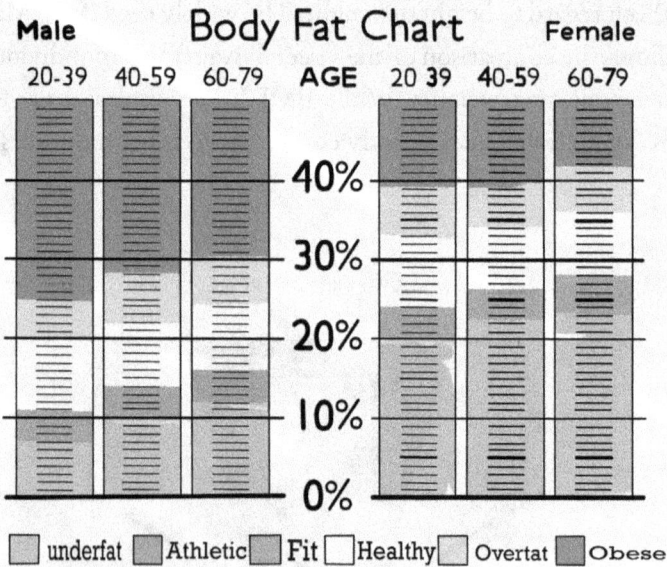

Example: For a Male 55 years old and a Fitness level of BMI=24.9,with Body Fat % between 19.9%, weight 169 .lb, Metabolic Age —44

Food Calorie Count

Evaluating the food you eat every day is necessary to achieve your health goals. Doing so will help you monitor your food intake in the future.

Calorie Intake Calculator: www.calculator.net/calorie-calculator.html

Calorie Calculator (Sample Results)

Gender	Male	
Age	55	
Height	5'-7"	
Weight	168 lbs. = 72Kg	Ideal weight 68 Kg = 168 Lbs.
Target Weight	149 lbs. = 68Kg	According to Height and Age
Activity	Activity Level 2	Sedentary or little activity
BMI	24.6	Healthy levels Below 25
Glucose at Fasting	128	Healthy Glucose 90-100

Calories Consumed a Day	Target	Action
2,183 calories a day	To maintain weight	Average American
1,683 calories a day	Lose 1 pound a week	Cut 500 calories a day
1,183 calories a day	Lose 2 pounds a week	Cut 1,000 calories a day
2,683 calories a day	Gain 1 pounds a week	Add 500 calories a day
3,183 calories a day	Gain 2 pounds a week	Add 1,000 calories a day
BMR – 1626 Cal/Day	TEE – 1989 Cal./Day	AEE- 460 Cal./Day

CALCULATING BURNED CALORIES

An easy way to find out how many calories you need to sustain your current weight and how many calories you need to burn to lose weight is by using the TANITA AM120E or a similar daily activity monitor that provides BMR, TEE, AEE, and Pedometer readings.

Sample of Calories burned:

Activity	Length of time	Calories Burned
Sitting	30 minutes	50
Walking (3 Miles/Hour)	30 minutes	280
Running (5 Miles / Hour)	30 minutes	430
Walking up Steps	30 minutes	450
Dancing	37 minutes	170
Sex	30 minutes	144
Bicycle	1 hour	200

Note: Actual values may vary depending on weight and sex and intensity levels. Each table/study of results may differ as conditions may be different. Verify your activity with corresponding tables from the web or consult with a professional trainer.

We emphasize the need to know your preferred activity and calories burned so you can balance your **Calories Equation**.

For a comprehensive table of activities, see Harvard Business School Chart: http://www.health.harvard.edu/newsweek/Calories-burned-in-30-minutes-of-leisure-and-routine-activities.htm

Total Body Water

The **percentage of water** in your body is directly related to muscle density. That is, the more fat you have in your body, the less water your body can hold. The more muscle in the body, the more water it can hold.

Average body water percentage ranges for healthy adults:
- Women: 44 to 60%
- Men: 50 to 66%

Drink four or more 8-ounce glasses of water every day to protect against development of high blood sugar (hyperglycemia). In a recent study, men and women with normal blood sugar levels who drank more than 34 ounces of water a day were 21% less likely to develop hyperglycemia over the next nine years than those who drank less than 16 ounces daily.

Basal Metabolic Rate (BMR) and Metabolic Age

Basal Metabolic Rate (BMR) is the amount of energy consumed per unit of time when your body is in neutral mode (sleeping, not moving), the digestive system is inactive, and energy expenditure is only sufficient to support normal functioning of the vital organs: the heart, lungs, nervous system, kidneys, liver, intestine, muscles, and skin. It takes about twelve hours of fasting to reach this state. Your basal rate is the number of calories you would burn if you stayed in bed all day.

Your **Metabolic Age** is calculated by comparing your BMR to the average BMR of your chronological age group. Formulas for calculating BMR take into account **age, weight, height, activity level, body fat, and lean body mass**.

The BMR Calculator – Use the TANITA AM120E or a similar device, or calculate the value yourself with the formula provided in this book (**Mifflin-St. Jeor equation**), or use the web to find a BMR calculator tool.

As we age, it becomes more difficult to eat whatever we want and stay slim, as the body's ability to burn energy slows with time. While your BMR decreases with age, depriving yourself of food in hopes of losing weight increases BMR, as the body needs energy. Regular aerobic exercise can increase BMR.

Body fat requires much less energy than lean muscle, which is more metabolically active and therefore requires more energy during activity. When comparing two individuals with all variables being equal, the person with more lean muscle mass will have a higher BMI and a lower metabolic age as that person's body requires more calories to muscle body.

Your **Metabolic Age** depends on how your BMR compares to others of the same chronological age. Metabolic age describes overall fitness and metabolic activity. **Metabolic age** is a reflection of physical health in the form of a calculation based on **BMR**. If one's metabolic age is lower than his actual age, it suggests that his body is in good health. A metabolic age higher than your chronological age indicates that you may be experiencing health problems. Be conscious, expand your awareness, and take action.

GLUCUT COACHING PROCESS

Results Time (Short-Term, Mid-Term, Long-Term)

The process of improving one's health depends on individual motivation. The GLUCUT COACHING program involves three key elements:

1. **BOOK** – Knowledge, Motivation, and Education – By reading this book you will come to understand what elements contribute to the status of your health and ready your mind for change.

2. **SELF-IMPROVEMENT PROCESS** –Take action after being educated and motivated

   • **Self-Assessment Checks** – Fill out the self-evaluation tables in this book, and consult with your healthcare provider to monitor your progress.

   • **Timetable Charts** – Continue with self-assessments as you change your lifestyle: 1-month, 6-month, and 1-year targets

   • **Food Modification Process** – Consult a dietician and build a diet with goals to achieve.

   • **Activity Modification Process** –Create a program and consult a healthcare professional to avoid drastic or negative health changes.

   • **Attend Personal Sessions** one-on-one with your GLUCUT Advisor in-person or via videoconference

3. **APP** – iPhone and Android smartphone application – A source for measuring tools, helpful reminders, and self-evaluation.

RESULTS

- **Short-term** (First month) – You will experience increased energy levels and stamina, and feel tired less often. You should see reduction in your daily glucose readings.

- **Mid-term** (2–6 months) – You should experience weight loss, slowly adjusting to your normal body/mass levels. BMI reduction will be noticeable. A1C will improve.

- **Long-term** (6 months and beyond) – You should see normal BMI levels for your age, height, build, and weight. You should feel much healthier overall with greater stamina and energy, mental and emotional wellbeing, and stable A1C readings. You will consume calories according to your body's needs in balance with your BMR and activity levels. You will likely eat smaller quantities of food, and will enjoy a sense of control over what you eat, the quantities you eat, and quality. Your metabolic age will improve to score below the average people in your segment. You will experience health improvements and monetary savings.

- **Embraced Lifestyle** – (3 years and up) You will know when the new way of life has become part of your routine when you make choices not because someone else tells you to, but because you believe they represent the most natural and comfortable way to live your life.

Goals and Measurements (statistics)

LIFE EXPECTANCY

As noted earlier, the average Japanese male lives to 80 years and the average woman lives to 86 years. They tend to live healthier longer, enjoy a more fruitful life, and are less likely to burden their supportive society. This level of longevity should be your personal target.

MEASUREMENTS INDICATING GOOD DIABETES MANAGEMENT

These THREE are often called the ABCs of diabetes:

1. **A1C** – blood sugar levels over the previous three months
2. **Blood pressure**
3. **Cholesterol Level** (LDL, HDL)

MEASUREMENTS INDICATING GOOD HEALTH MANAGEMENT

Here are seven GLUCUT Coaching Indicators based on: **Weight, Height, Age, Activity Levels, and Body Composition**

- **BMI**
- **BMR** – Basal Metabolic Rate (Minimum calories needed for Survival)
- **Caloric Intake**—TEE
- **Metabolic Age**
- **Body Fat**
- **Visceral Fat**
- **MET** – Intensity of Daily Activity levels (1.2 Sedentary – 1.55 Active Exercise, Harris Benedict Formula), the more active you are the higher the number.

When your measurements fall outside healthy ranges for any of these indicators, you are more likely to be burdened by complications of Pre-Diabetes and Diabetes Type 2, which may include **heart disease, stroke, kidney disease, blindness, and even amputation in worst case scenarios**. Take action. Motivate yourself to make permanent change that will result in incredible personal transformation.

Even if you don't experience extreme diabetic symptoms, you may still suffer from: low capacity to move, fatigue, light sensitivity, bad skin, clogging, leg cramps, low appetite, erectile dysfunction, fluctuating emotional state (edginess, depression, sadness, etc).

Gradual deterioration of the body is often not noticed until too late. Damaged health does not happen in one day; neither will it disappear in a short time. What takes years to develop will take years to correct. Every organism in nature adapts to new conditions; our bodies adapt to bad blood conditions and try to survive. In the same way, your body will adjust to new conditions, and revert back to a healthy state given sufficient effort and time.

A study by the **National Institute of Health** shows a significant improvement in diabetes control directly related to managing the measures listed above. Not only does this study validate the importance of these measures with respect to diabetes management, it also validates the principles of GLUCUT COACHING.

Source: Data from Columbia University (New York) & Tanita Institute (Tokyo)

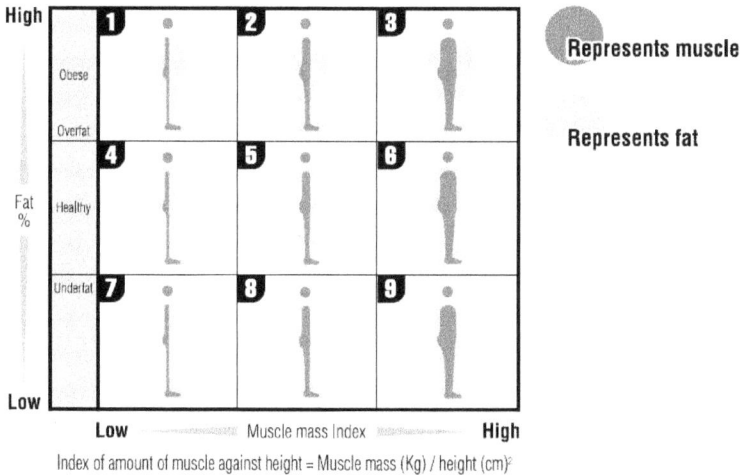

Index of amount of muscle against height = Muscle mass (Kg) / height (cm)²

GLUCUT COACHING PROCESS

Short and Long Term Savings

You will realize extensive savings as a result of participating in the GLU-CUT COACHING program. You will spend less on medical expenses, food, and alcohol. And although you do pay for GLUCUT COACHING, the amount of money you will save (not to mention the health benefits) far outweighs the program's cost.

The main long-term health benefits you will get from GLUCUT COACHING include significant reduction of healthcare costs. On average, a person with type 2 diabetes spends around $1,000 each month on medical expenses. According to the Center for Decease Control, the annual healthcare cost for a person with diabetes in the US (in 2009) was $11,700. Compare that figure to the average for a person without diabetes: $4,400 (Includes Medicine and Insurance).

Calculated Savings

MEDECINE SAVINGS

Assume one can save 50% in pharmaceutical (Medicine) expenses. Based on 2009 prices: ($11,700 − $4,400)/2 (50%) = $3,650/year x 20 years = $73,000 Savings (The cost of 2 mid-sized luxury sedans). Adjusted to inflation in 2014 ($4,050/year) = $81,000.

Age of Diabetes Diagnosis to Death	Total years x Savings (2010 prices)	Total Medicine Savings
55 to 75	20 Years x $4,050 a year	$81,000
50 to 75	25 Years x $4,050 a year	$101,250
45 to 75	30 Years x $4,050 a year	$121,500
40 to 75	35 Years x $4,050 a year	$141,750
35 to 75	40 Years x $4,050 a year	$162,000
30 to 75	45 Years x $4,050 a year	$182,250

Calculations for different age groups consider a life expectancy of 75 years (in 2010 Prices): The savings are significant for all age groups.

The U.S. Bureau of Labor Statistics monitors employment, inflation, average pay, and benefits, as well as consumer spending. In 2009, they found that the average American spent $6,443 annually on food. In 2014 prices, that is $7.

Food Savings

Assume you can save 25% of your food consumption by eating fewer calories. Subtract $1,785.50 a year from a total consumption of $7,150 a year

Age for Saving	Years x Savings	Food Savings
55 to 75	20 x $1,785.50	$35,710
50 to 75	25 x $1,785.50	$44,627
45 to 75	30 x $1,785.50	$53,565
40 to 75	35 x $1,785.50	$62,492
35 to 75	40 x $1,785.50	$75,020
30 to 75	45 x $1,785.50	$80,347

Savings: Medecine + Food

Assuming a reduction only of 25% in costs:

Age for Saving	Years x Savings	Savings
55 to 75	20 x $4,237.50	$116,710
50 to 75	25 x $4,237.50	$145,877

45 to 75	30 x $4,237.50	$175,065
40 to 75	35 x $4,237.50	$204,242
35 to 75	40 x $4,237.50	$237,020
30 to 75	45 x $4,237.50	$263,597

These savings equal the average cost of a house in the US in 2014.

MONITORING COSTS

Costs of monitoring program:

$30/Month (average) x 12 = $365/year x 3 years = $1,095 (entire program cost).

Monitoring Costs Year	GLUCUT COACHING Yearly Costs	Yearly Savings Medicine + Food
1	$365	$5,077.50
2	$365	$5,077.50
3	$365	$5,077.50
TOTAL	$1,095	$15,232.50

It is important to note that you will most likely need to follow the program for the rest of your life, not just for 3 years, to maintain the level of savings shown above. However, once you have followed the program for 3 years, you will have developed a strong and reliable routine to follow for years to come with little to no outside assistance.

STORE

Through our online store, you can purchase items you won't find elsewhere:

Books

Food Book (Japanese book and 500 Cal Diet Recipes) Amazon

Accessories

Tanita Weight Scale (Weight, Body Fat, Bone Mass, Calories) Amazon

Tanita/OMRON – Pedometer (Pacer) Amazon

Tea/Water Thermos – Amazon

Massage Chair—Panasonic

Food

Supplements and Distinctive Japanese foods, sweets, teas, and others.

Ceramics/Home Accessories

Ceramics sets/ Home accessories (Size Plate and Bento Box) Yukiko

Cosmetics

Cosmetics (Natural body cleansing) Amazon

Travel

Travel (Onsen and Ryokan, nature base)

Furniture

Japanese Wood original furniture

Design (Architecture/Buildings/Interiors)

Natural Wood base – renewable materials- Japanese site

Clothes

Clothes / Accessories (100% cotton natural and loose outfit) Amazon

SUPPORTING ARTICLES and RECOMMENDED READING

"American Diet Report Card," *Center for Science in the Public Interest*, 2013

"Checking Your Blood Glucose," *American Diabetes Association*, 2014.

"Drinking Water May Cut Risk of High Blood Sugar," Catherine Laino, *WebMD Health News*, 2011.

"Employers measure workers' waistlines," *CNN Money*, October 17, 2014

"How Stress Affects Diabetes," *American Diabetes Association*, 2013.

Matvienko, Oksana A., and James D. Hoehns. "A lifestyle intervention study in patients with diabetes or impaired glucose tolerance: translation of a research intervention into practice." *The Journal of the American Board of Family Medicine*, 2009.

"Mental Health," *American Diabetes Association*, 2014.

"National Institute of Health study shows big improvement in diabetes control over past decades," February, 2013.

"Obese lose up to eight years of life," James Gallagher, *BBC News*. December 2014.

"The Story of the Human Body: Evolution, Health, and Disease," Daniel Lieberman, *Harvard University*, 2013.

"What Does a 1,500-Calorie Diet Look Like?," *Eatingwell.com*, 2010.

"Years of life lost and healthy life-years lost from diabetes and cardiovascular disease in overweight and obese people: a modeling study," Grover et al. *The Lancet*, December 2014.

Additional information: http://www.diabetes.org/living-with-diabetes/complications/mental-health/#sthash.cIlNFdm0.dpuf

PERSONAL NOTES

We recommend using this section to list your short, mid, and long term goals.

_____

_____

_____

_____

_____

_____

_____

_____

_____

_____

_____

_____

_____

_____

_____

_____

_____

_____

_____

www.ingramcontent.com/pod-product-compliance
Lightning Source LLC
Chambersburg PA
CBHW070813290326
41931CB00011BB/2205